Microscopic Analysis of the Anastomoses between the Cranial Nerves

Microscopic Analysis of the Anastomoses between the Cranial Nerves

by Ernst Philipp Eduard Bischoff, M.D.
translated and edited by Ernest Sachs, Jr., M.D.
and Eva W. Valtin

University Press of New England Hanover, New Hampshire 1977

Library of Congress Catalogue Card Number 77-72520
International Standard Book Number 0-87451-143-7
Printed in the United States of America

The University Press of New England

Sponsoring Institutions:

Brandeis University
Clark University
Dartmouth College
University of New Hampshire
University of Rhode Island
University of Vermont

Contents

Legends and figures may be found on the following pages:

Background of Bischoff's Monograph

BY ERNEST SACHS, JR., M.D.

The existence of anastomoses between the cranial nerves is a subject most neurologists, neurosurgeons, and otolaryngologists today do not consider. Yet for well over one hundred years connections between the trigeminal, facial, vestibular, glossopharyngeal, vagus, spinal accessory, hypoglossal, and upper cervical nerves have been known.

Ernst Philipp Bischoff, a young doctor working in his father's Anatomical Institute in Munich, carried out an extraordinarily detailed piece of anatomical research in 1863–64. This scholarly research was done in response to a prize competition offered by the Royal Medical Faculty of Munich on the subject of "Anastomosis between the Cranial Nerves." Bischoff's thesis won the award, which was announced on June 26, 1864. The work was published in Munich in 1865 in a fifty-two page monograph, accompanied by 109 precise drawings of his magnified dissections. This exact and scrupulously honest piece of work has been virtually disregarded, in fact lost to the neurological world, for over one hundred years.

In his dissections Bischoff took great pains to use acetic acid and the dissecting microscope to help clarify the difference between nerves, connective tissue, and small vessels. The reader will do well to study his careful explanations in the section on method. Bischoff usually used dissecting loupes of from 3 to 12 power, and rechecked his findings with a dissecting microscope up to 50X. With the Dujardin prism he was able to trace his magnified dissections directly.

I have been able to find no reference to the study in any anatomy book, not even in the old German textbooks of anatomy by Toldt and by Sabotta. The first edition of Sabotta was published in Wurzburg in May 1906. I first became aware of the existence of Bischoff's work from the bibliography in White and Sweet, *Pain, Its Mechanisms and Neurosurgical Control* while searching for an explanation of some observations I had made in patients I had operated on in 1952. They had had severe unilateral face and head pain involving the ear. Reasoning that there might be some involvement of the nervus intermedius of Wrisberg, previously described by J. Ramsey

Hunt, L. T. Furlow, A. A. Wilson, D. Cooper and D. Cavicke, and others, I sectioned the nervus intermedius in both patients, who have been relieved of their pain until the present day (1976).

Operating with 2½ power magnifying loupes at a time before the surgical microscope was familiar to neurosurgeons, I observed some unusual connections between the nervus intermedius and the 7th and 8th cranial nerves which were not described in any anatomy books. I published these observations in 1968. After learning of Bischoff's monograph in White and Sweet's bibliography, I searched the medical libraries and anatomy books throughout this country and abroad for a copy. None could be found. It was then that I learned through the kindness of Dr. William Sweet, Professor of Neurological Surgery at Harvard, that he had found a copy of Bischoff's monograph in an obscure second-hand medical book store! He kindly lent it to me for study and copying. To my knowledge, this is one of the few copies in existence.*

For many years I sought a German-English scholar sufficiently versed, willing, and able to translate the rather awkward, clumsy, neuroanatomical German of the 1860s. Not until I met Mrs. Eva W. Valtin of Washington, D.C., mother of my physiology colleague Professor Heinz Valtin of the Dartmouth Medical School and an official translator for the National Medical Library, did I find anyone scholarly enough to make the translation. Mrs. Valtin lived in Germany from 1896 to 1938 before coming to the United States and has had extensive experience in translating German to English and English to German. She studied at a number of German universities; she has had considerable experience in medical translating. Though not a neuroanatomist, her translation of Bischoff's work is meticulous and precise; together we coped with the changes in the nomenclature of nerves which have occurred over the past 111 years, as well as typographical errors, abbreviations, and enormously complex sentences! To make the work readable we have taken slight liberties in translation, but have been careful never to change Bischoff's actual observations or opinions.

Bischoff's thesis, he says in his preface, was criticized by his professors on two counts. One was that he did not include a summary at the end. He corrected this in the published version. The other was that he made no references to his figures or legends in his text, saving all the illustrations and then all the legends until the end of the monograph! He reasoned that it would break up the text and make it "too cumbersome and too involved." We disagree; the

*One copy is listed in the Surgeon General's Library, Pamphlet Collection 305, Vol. 1, A–L, p. 159 (1873); one in the Munich Medical Library; and one in the Countway Library at Harvard.

illustrations and legends are an indispensable part of the work, and I have therefore taken great pains to insert them at the places where the findings are being discussed and described.

Bischoff, in the manner of his day, referred to over forty authors but gave no bibliography. I have created one in which I have looked up all the references and have either found them or found something about the authors. I have also added editorial comments at places where Bischoff has been corroborated or not, and where an explanation seemed in order.

I am deeply indebted to Mrs. Valtin for helping me to bring this monograph to the attention of the English speaking world and indeed the twentieth-century world of neural science. I am grateful to the Hitchcock Foundation for a grant to help defray expenses. I am particularly indebted to Dr. William Sweet, who made available to me one of the few copies of this monograph in existence.

Hanover, New Hampshire
1976

Ernest Sachs, Jr., M.D.

Mikroskopische Analyse

der

Anastomosen der Kopfnerven.

Gekrönte Beantwortung

der

von der königlich medizinischen Fakultät zu München im Jahre 1863
ausgesetzten Preisfrage

durch

Ernst Philipp Eduard Bischoff,
Dr. Med.

Mit dreiundvierzig Steindrucktafeln.

München, 1865.
Verlag der J. J. Lentner'schen Buchhandlung.
(E. Stahl.)

Microscopic Analysis
of the
Anastomoses between the Cranial Nerves

Award Winning Answer
to
the special problem proposed for competition by the
Royal Medical Faculty of Munich in the year 1863
by

Ernst Philipp Eduard Bischoff, M.D.

---

with 43 lithographs

Munich 1865
J. J. Leutner Bookstore, Publisher
(E. Stahl)

Preface

I am taking the liberty of submitting to the world of science this paper, which has been written as an answer to the special problem proposed by the medical faculty of the University of Munich for the year 1863–64. This paper has been awarded the first prize, and I venture to publish herewith the citation, which is extremely flattering and was made public in an open session of the faculty on June 26, 1864:

> The contestant in the competition concerning "Microscopic Analysis of the Cranial Nerves" has arrived with great aptitude at the answer to this problem, which required a thorough preparation of the anatomical-microscopic models which could only be accomplished with skillful hands. He has evaluated his numerous experiments with vision and with recognition of prior studies. He is, therefore, awarded the first prize.

In the review of my paper, the consultant has voiced two reservations which I would like to justify at this point. The first one was that in the text I did not refer to the respective figures. I did not do so because I was afraid that if I acted as suggested, the text might become cumbersome and too involved. I believe that my method makes it easy for anatomists and physicians familiar with neurology (the only ones who will be interested in my paper) to understand what I have to say, even without pointing out the figures. I have added to the pictures explanations that are as exact as possible.

The second criticism dealt with the fact that I had neglected to give a short summary of the entire paper. This was an oversight due to the short time available, and I will certainly add a summary to the present form of the paper.

Finally, may I be permitted to mention that because of his indispensable material and resources, I could not avoid enlisting the knowledge and participation of my father as the chairman of the Institute of Anatomy, who for that reason declined to be a member of the reviewing panel. Without my father's cooperation and that of his associate Dr. Rudiger, I could not have undertaken a study of such magnitude which required great experience in anatomy. I would like, therefore, to express publicly my gratitude and deep appreciation to these two gentlemen.

I hope this work will find approval within the wider circle of scientists beyond those I know and esteem.

The paper will appear without changes in the form in which it was submitted to the faculty.

Munich
October 1, 1865

Ernst Philipp Eduard Bischoff

Introduction

I have ventured to follow the invitation of the esteemed medical faculty and have undertaken a microscopic analysis of the better known anastomoses of the cranial nerves. I am submitting herewith the results of my studies to the faculty for their judgment.

From the outset I was well aware of the great difficulties that had to be overcome, and this fact became more and more evident, the further the work progressed. Indeed, no expert will doubt that technically the dissection of the cranial nerves is one of the most difficult anatomical undertakings; I had believed that the analysis of the prepared nerves would in fact be much easier and simpler than it actually turned out to be.

I therefore appeal to the indulgence of the faculty. Although I trust that I have succeeded in explaining certain rather interesting facts regarding the nature of the cranial nerves, I am well aware that quite a few other points are still dubious. Time was of the essence, however, and often I had to refrain from repeating the study of some of the nerves.

The Method Used

For the usual preparations of the respective nerve segments, I used heads of adults as well as of new born children which had been preserved in wine spirits. When it was a question—as was usually the case—of breaking off bones and opening up bony channels, I used hammer and chisel and bone forceps in the case of bones softened by acid, and not a knife, as did Beck and some others. In certain cases Beck's method has possible advantages; it seemed to me, however, that the disadvantages caused by changes or even destruction to which delicate nerves are exposed when they lie in strong acids for a prolonged period of time far outweigh those advantages; practice and experience have taught me that my own method is less likely to lead to a failure in the study of even a very complicated nerve segment. For some experiments with particularly delicate branching of nerves, I wetted the area under study with acetic acid in order that the delicate nerves would appear more clearly and not be endangered when they were completely exposed and lifted out. Without being cleared completely, they were then separated with great care; otherwise delicate fibers, which can only be detected with the help of a very considerable magnification, might be cut away; they often contain the answer to the apparent anastomosis. On the other hand, not too much of the surrounding connective tissue must be left on the nerves, since that might cause the preparation to appear unclear under the magnifying glass or the microscope.

After the preparation was separated and lifted out, it was immediately spread exactly in its original position on a colored wax tablet or on a slide. The former procedure was employed when additional work with knife and scissors was needed; if necessary this was done under a tripod magnifying glass with an enlargement of from five to ten times, often after the preparation had been cleared by means of acetic acid. Since this enlargement enabled me to detect even the most delicate and small nerve fibers because of their white color, this was the safest way to recognize the relative position and connection of two nerves. But even when I put the preparation immediately on a slide, I first spread it with two pins under the magnifying glass and tried to detect right away the relationship of the nerves to each other.

After the preparation had been laid out in its natural position, I added a few drops of a rather weak acetic acid solution in order to make it lighter and to facilitate the recognition of the nerves. The acid soon makes the connective tissue transparent and translucent, while the nerves, particularly those of the brain and the spinal cord, and less so the sympathetic nerves, the thicker sides of which also become transparent, remain white; thus I could be sure that I would not confuse vessels or fibers of the connective tissue with nerves. Acetic acid serves this purpose perfectly, completely, and quickly not only for fresh preparations but also for those that were repeatedly submerged in water or had been preserved in wine spirits. Unfortunately, however, acetic acid also causes the preparation to shrink or to swell, and this makes certain findings unclear.

I took pains to prevent that from happening by carefully pressing the preparation, either by putting a piece of glass on top of it or by means of a compressor. This manipulation is essential and important, for it helps to spread the preparation, clears it up completely, and with a strong enlargement makes it suitable for study even under the microscope. In order to obtain the correct position of the nerves or to be able to change the position for the purpose of a more exact discovery of certain points, I sometimes tied a fine thread to single nerves, with the help of which and by creating a mild compression, I could tighten and draw them to and fro. In the case of thicker nerves—as for instance the orbital nerves at their point of entrance into the orbit through the superior orbital fissure, the sphenopalatine ganglion, the facial nerve, etc.—the use of compression frequently gets to be very difficult, because the nerve retracts and slides away. When that happened, I rendered the nerve segment as thin as possible and cut out a little piece, in order to create the compression.

As extremely useful and indispensable as the compression may be, however, it is dangerous, and I cannot advise strongly enough that it be used with extreme care. It can happen too easily that one nerve is covered by another one, or that one nerve runs on top of the other, and the compression might make it appear that they connect. This occurs particularly when the nerves run in different planes or are very closely interlaced. In such cases the difficulties are very great, and only repeated experiments and changes of position can protect against errors.

Another method used for the detection of certain conditions and of the connections and ramifications of certain nerves consisted in the stripping of the nerve sheath; here the treatment with acetic acid as described above was also very useful, for it causes the sheath to swell and to separate from the nerve, thus making it easier to split the sheath and pull it off. This method has often served especially well for the study of the facial nerves. Here, too, however, one must beware of errors, since it can very easily happen that a small nerve strand gets torn off, so that it seems not to exist or not to be connected. It is therefore necessary to watch out for the direction the little branch takes in relation to the main trunk. Whenever possible, I performed this operation using a loupe, so that I could observe exactly what happened.

In some cases where the presence of fat greatly hindered recognition of the situation, as when examining the sphenopalatine and the otic ganglion, I have treated the preparation with ether. After it had been submerged for some time in a stronger acetic acid, in which the fatty cells are usually dissolved, I submerged it in ether and allowed the fat to be drawn out; thus the preparation very often became much lighter.

After the preparation had been well spread out and cleared up under the loupe with a three-, five-, or twelvefold magnification, I proceeded to sketch it with the help of a Dujardin prism. I cannot say often enough how much aid I derived from this procedure. Through it I saved a tremendous amount of time and there was no other way to assure that the sketches were correct with regard to the relative thickness and length of the nerves. The outlines were usually drafted within a few minutes, but even the most skillful draftsman applying a much greater effort could not have done a better job.* In addition I was able, while I was drawing, to pursue all details and to follow up every fiber with my pencil.

When the first drawing was sketched, using a moderate enlargement, I placed the preparation under a microscope in order to examine the details of the connections between the individual nerve twigs and branches and if necessary to correct the drawing. Here I rarely needed an enlargement above fifty times. Only if it was a case of recognizing extremely fine fibers to be nerves and of distinguishing them from vessels, or of determining the kind of nerves—whether they were coarser or finer, cerebral or sympathetic nerves—only then did I use stronger magnification. It seems hardly necessary to mention that it is usually not difficult to distinguish nerves from vessels under the microscope, particularly when the preparation has been made lighter with acetic acid. The transverse and circular fibers which every little vessel that is not extremely thin possesses make it very easy to distinguish them from nerves.

With the degree of enlargement I have used in the drawings only a portion of the nerve could be shown. Only the microscope gives an exact picture. This should not be regarded as a mistake; otherwise the size of the drawings would have been enormous.

Finally, I have tried to preserve the preparations. For this purpose the acetic acid was washed out with water; then I placed the preparation under moderate pressure in the correct position between two glass plates and dropped them into strong wine spirits. After they had lain in the alcohol for some time and had hardened, I let them imbibe as much as necessary in carmine acid ammonia. After that, they were again compressed between two glass plates, in pure alcohol, and finally either in a shellac solution or in Canada balsam, which had been dissolved in ether. Thus they became lighter, and it was quite easy to observe the position of the nerves under the loupe or the microscope, since the nerves had imbibed a lot while the surrounding connective tissues had done so to a far lesser degree. Unfortunately, however, it was extremely difficult to avoid air bubbles during treatment with Canada balsam, for rather delicate nerves became brittle in the pure alcohol and were twisted and sometimes even torn. Preserved preparations are therefore much less valuable than fresh ones, especially in view of the fact that they cannot easily be observed from all sides. Consequently, they serve mainly as confirmation of the drawings.

Having outlined the general method of my study, I will now proceed to the description of the individual anastomoses; in doing so I will in each case relate the special method I used.

But first I would like to make a few remarks.

*[Such modesty! *Ed.*]

The So-Called Nerve Anastomoses in General

In view of our present knowledge of the exact structure of the nerves and their composition of primitive fibers or tubes, it seems clear that we cannot speak of a true nerve anastomosis; it differs from a vessel anastomosis, which signifies a genuine connection. [Bischoff takes pains to explain that the nerve anastomoses he is describing consist of fibers leaving one nerve trunk and *joining the course of another nerve.* He hastens to explain that the axones do not physically join, as blood vessels may. In present day parlance, there would be no possibility of axoplasmic flow from one nerve to another. *Ed.*] The primitive sheath of the nerves never connects, and in this sense the name "nerve anastomosis" has lost its meaning. It signifies either a changed association of the nerve fibers or a union of various nerves by means of a ganglion. Only in recent years has this manner of connection become known. We now understand that the so-called ganglia consist of an accumulation of ganglion cells, and that nerves exist in their midst. The relationship of the two elements in the ganglia to each other is still unknown. Although some scientists are convinced that the projections detected on the ganglia are directly connected with the nerves and that such connections have actually been observed, many factors that would establish the general validity of these findings are still missing; it has not even been proven that all ganglion cells have such projections which connect them with nerves. It is conceivable, however, that such ganglia could affect a connection between nerve sheaths belonging to different nerves, thus representing a new and true kind of nerve anastomosis. We shall see that there is reason to believe that such anastomoses effected by ganglia do indeed exist at special points along the cranial nerves.

Although recognition of the pseudo-nerve anastomoses has lost its validity as far as a genuine connection of nerves is concerned, it is physiologically important to determine the position of the different nerves next to each other in varying sequence as well as their peripheral extension; in that manner the same part can receive elements belonging to different nerves. Such new association of the fibers of two nerves can be a mutual exchange (Hyrtl), or just unilateral connection. In the first case, there is a mutual exchange of fibers which may be permanent or temporary—"anastomosis temporanea"; in the latter case, the fibers return to their own nerves, or they join another nerve. [Sachs; Saunders and Sachs]

Of particular interest—although enigmatic—would be a kind of nerve anastomosis which as far as I know was first pointed out by Volkmann and more recently by Hyrtl, and which has been named a "regressive anastomosis" or "nerves without end." Volkmann (*Müller's Archiv,* 1840, p. 510) believed that he had found in humans, and also in some animals, anastomoses between various nerves, where nerves pass from one to another and return centrally without extending at the periphery. This was supposed to happen in the case of the trochlear nerve and the ophthalmic nerve in the calf, between the second and third cervical nerves, and the spinal accessory in the well known ansa hypoglossi between the descending ramus of this nerve and the second and the third cervical nerves and also between the second and the third cervical nerves themselves.

Hyrtl (*Natural History Review,* January 1862, p. 96) has also called attention to those anastomoses and in addition has pointed out several other examples: anastomoses between the right and the left hypoglossal nerves in the muscular part of the geniohyoid; between the hypoglossal nerve and the anterior ramus of the first cervical nerve; between the loops of the anterior rami of the spinal nerves; between the nerves of the plantar and the palmar arch of the foot and the hand; between an accessory obturator nerve, in case it exists, and the genuine obturator nerve.

Since these nerve anastomoses—if they really exist—are completely enigmatic as far as our knowledge is concerned (and the only possible explanation could be that in their strange peripheral course they bring about the connection between two central parts), I have paid particular attention to them in the area where they affect my study.

It is obvious that great caution must be employed, for the nerve fibers, whose curved course seems to travel from one nerve to another and return the same way, may possibly take a peripheral route through very small strands that cannot be detected with the naked eye, or they may be hidden by nerves that branch off at a higher level. Volkmann has repudiated Kronenberg's assumption of such retrograde nerves at the uniting angle of the anterior and posterior roots of the spinal nerves, because the sensory function of the anterior roots—detected by Magendie—stops when one cuts into the angle to a depth of ½"!* He saw that not a loop but a crossing of the two roots is formed; this fact completely explains the success of Kronenberg's experiment.

I am now more or less convinced that at certain spots where it was believed that such retrograde nerves were found, a peripheral ramification had taken place instead, and that an error had been committed. Even if I have not succeeded completely, I did see, nevertheless, that the primary fibers in order to reach their periph-

*[Bischoff uses the symbol ½"! We have not been able to determine with certainty what this symbol means, but feel sure on anatomical grounds that it must mean ½ mm. *Ed.*]

eral extension take such a complicated and strange course that it seems unwarranted to deny their existence entirely even at places where it cannot be found and proven. Therefore, I must express my doubts in regard to the "nerves without end," insofar as I was able to examine them. [These probably *do* exist, and mean simply loop connections. *Ed.*]

I. The Upper Three Sensory Nerves*

At this time it is still doubtful whether and in what manner an anastomosis exists between any of the first three sensory nerves and any other nerve. There is certainly none with the olfactory nerve, nor does a junction between the optic nerve and the sphenopalatine ganglion—first pointed out by Hirzel (*Zeitschrift f. Phys.,* I, p. 228)—represent a true anastomosis, although other anatomists, e.g. Arnold, Valentin, Krause, believed that they had detected it. What they assumed to be a genuine anastomosis, however, is in fact a thread of the ganglion belonging to the sheath of the optic nerve.

Chaussier, Ribes, Kusel, Hirzel, and, in particular, Tiedemann believed they saw connections between the optic nerve and the ciliary nerves and the ciliary ganglion when they described delicate tiny nerve strands originating from those nerves or ganglia; these presumably reach the retina together with the central artery of the retina and the short posterior ciliary arteries. According to Arnold (*Anatomie,* II, p. 970), a small strand also runs to the retina from the internal carotid plexus with the central artery of the retina.

Although these statements are found repeatedly in almost all manuals and textbooks, it seems that only Beck specifically examined these nerves *Über die Verbindung des Sehn-nerven mit dem Augen- und Nasen knoten,* Heidelberg, 1847). After multitudes of experiments, he denied the existence of those connections in humans and animals, while Arnold (*Anatomie,* II, p. 888) leaves their existence in doubt. Anyway, they would have to be regarded as connections with the sympathetic nerves and not as [true cranial nerve—*ed.*] anastomoses and therefore do not concern my study.

Scientists speak with great certainty about anastomoses between the auditory nerve and the facial nerve within the internal auditory meatus. Wrisberg, Kollner, Scarpa, Breschet, Swan, Arnold, Varrentrapp, Lauth, Cruveillhier, Beck, Krause, Valentin, Hyrtl, Bock, and many others say that they have observed such an anastomosis.

*[It will be noted that Bischoff after describing the olfactory and optic nerves discusses the nervus intermedius of Wrisberg VII and VIII before discussing the trigeminal. *Ed.*]

On the other hand, Haller, Sommering, and Longet (*Anat. d. Nerven-systems,* übers. von Hein, II, p. 350) say that its existence is an illusion. Arnold and Valentin have given the most detailed descriptions. According to them, there is a double anastomosis, namely first an inner one (communicating ramus internus) which belongs to the lesser root or the nervus intermedius and consists of one or more thin threads; these run in the internal auditory canal from the facial nerve to the vestibular portion of the auditory nerve (sometimes even before they enter the canal) [Sachs, 1968]. The second one is an external anastomosis (communicating ramus externus) which consists of a single or a double—usually very delicate—thread between the vestibular portion of the auditory and the genu of the facial nerve, and apparently is connected with the greater as well as lesser superficial petrosal (Arnold, *Anatomie,* I, p. 865). It seems that Arnold regards it as related to the sympathetic system, in which case it would go from the petrosal to the facial and from there to the auditory nerve. Valentin (*Hirn und Nervenlehre,* p. 441) says that the major part of the latter goes from the auditory to the facial nerve and the smaller part from the facial, or better from both petrosal nerves, to the auditory nerve.

In each of twenty-seven cases studied, Beck (*Anat. Unters. über d. VII. u. IX. Hirnnervenpaar,* p. 25) found the anastomosis, but usually in its single form, passing from fibers of the facial to the acoustic nerve or vice versa. He believes the junction to be of no importance inasmuch as it represents only the separation of the rootlets of both nerves, which because of their origin close to each other does not become complete until their destination has been reached.

Sappey (*Anatomie,* II, p. 252) describes the apparent anastomosis as being mediated by Wrisberg's nervus intermedius; presumably it consists of two fibers, one of which at first seems to lie next to the acoustic, the other one next to the facial nerve, after which they join and form a small ramus, thus giving the appearance of an anastomosis. Incidentally, this nervus intermedius is said to join the ramus of the facial nerve through two delicate threads at the beginning of the canal of Fallopius and only at the end totally combines with the geniculate ganglion.

It might be assumed that the answer to this question would not present great difficulties, since the preparation of the involved part of the nerve seems to be relatively simple. It is mandatory, however, to remove with extreme caution the part of the brain where the two nerves originate, because roots of the auditory nerve and the nervus intermedius are so soft that the latter may easily be torn off. For an accurate study the connection of the origin with the particular part of the brain must be absolutely intact. Furthermore, the genu of the facial nerve must be chiseled out, and the two rami of the auditory nerve, especially the vestibular ramus, has to be severed close to the entrance into the labyrinth. The examination of the preparation itself, which is not at all easy, must be carried out even more carefully. At the outset one must guard against mistaking for anastomoses vascular branches which extend between the two nerves and the nervus intermedius. Great care has to be taken in the separation of those vessels around the roots of the nerves, in order not to tear apart tiny nerves whose observation is essential. Furthermore, the ramification of the nervus intermedius is so complicated that very special attention must be paid to its course. I do not understand how Beck could describe these facts as being simple, and I for one, wonder whether he really examined them. Nor is Sappey's description exact, although he comes closer to the truth. In any case, Arnold is right in stating that it is absolutely necessary to explore both [the VII and VIII] nerves in connection with their central origin. I did it more than once, and although the connection between the two nerves brought about by the nervus intermedius appears very different when scrutinized, I agree with Arnold and Valentin that it is a double one, namely—as Arnold has called it—an inner and an outer one, since one connection occurs during their course in the internal auditory meatus and the other connection at the very end of the auditory canal between the facial and the vestibular nerve. I am convinced, however, that these connections are not anastomoses in the true sense of the word, namely that nerve fibers of one nerve completely merge with the course of another nerve; this particular anastomosis is not a genuine one, since the two threads separate again after they have joined. As said before, it is Wrisberg's nervus intermedius that brings about the anastomoses [Figures 1-8]. The latter is generally regarded as belonging to the facial nerve; but I want to emphasize that in regard to the origin of the fibers it is hard to draw a definite conclusion, for they are in evidence partly close to and alongside the facial nerve, and partly close to and together with the acoustic nerve. Yet some of them are joined permanently with the vestibular nerve. On the way they bring about a junction of the facial with the acoustic nerve and the other way around. I think that it is this change which justifies my denial of a genuine transition of the fibers of one nerve to the other. Such would indeed be quite unbelievable anyway. [See *ed.* comment above, page 9.] I say the same in regard to the so-called outer connection which occurs at the very back of the auditory canal by means of several extremely delicate small threads, although I am aware of the fact that—if one accomplishes the separation with great caution and care—its repeated appearance seems very strange. Here, too, the fibers

FIGURES 1 TO 8

The anastomosis between facial and auditory nerve. All figures show that the apparent anastomosis is produced by the fibers of Wrisberg's nervus intermedius going back and forth between auditory and facial nerve. This nerve is usually regarded as belonging to the facial nerve. An exact study of the figures shows, however, that this is impossible, since the fibers just as often originate from the acoustic nerve as from the merger with the facial nerve or from the space between the two. Therefore, I have decided that the segment that definitely stays with the facial nerve belongs to this nerve from the start, and the same applies to the segment that definitely merges with the acoustic—to which it must be considered as belonging from the beginning.

The meaning of the letters is as follows:

a facial nerve

b auditory nerve

c fibers of the nervus intermedius

d genu of the facial nerve and the origin of the greater superficial petrous

[Note errors in Figures 5 and 7, in which "a" and "b" are reversed and wrongly label the facial and auditory nerves. *Ed.*]

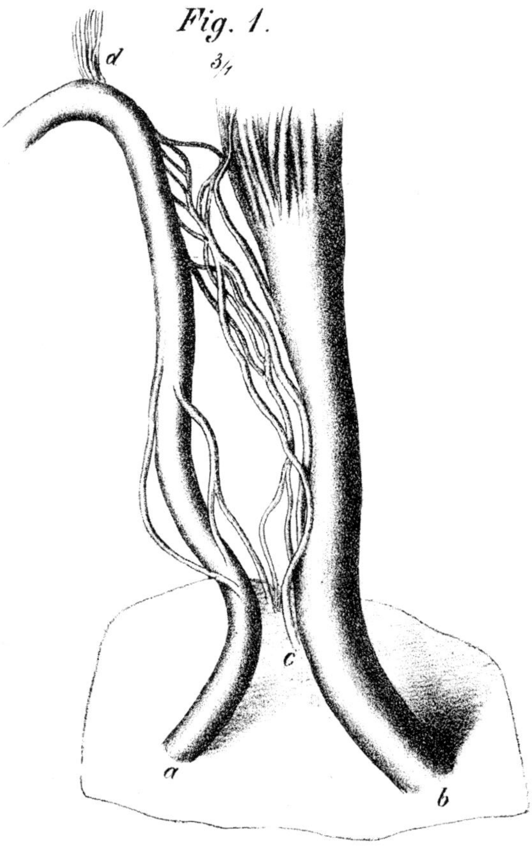

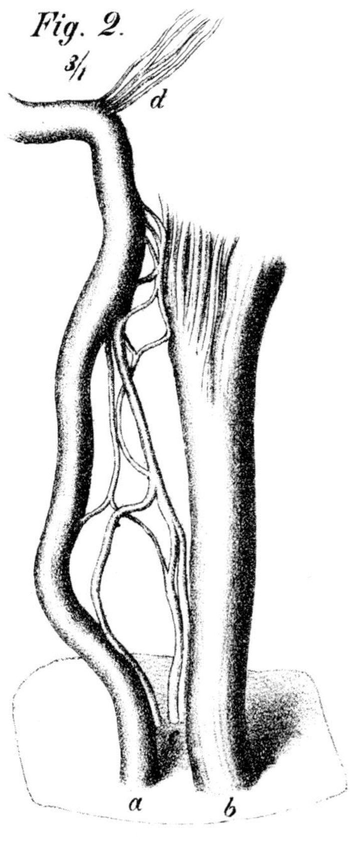

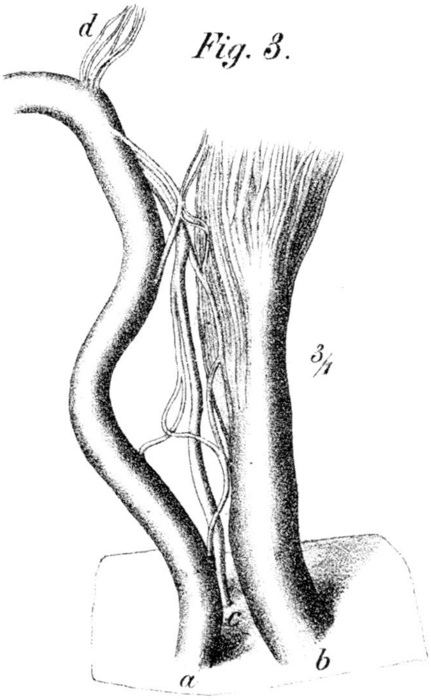

Fig. 3.

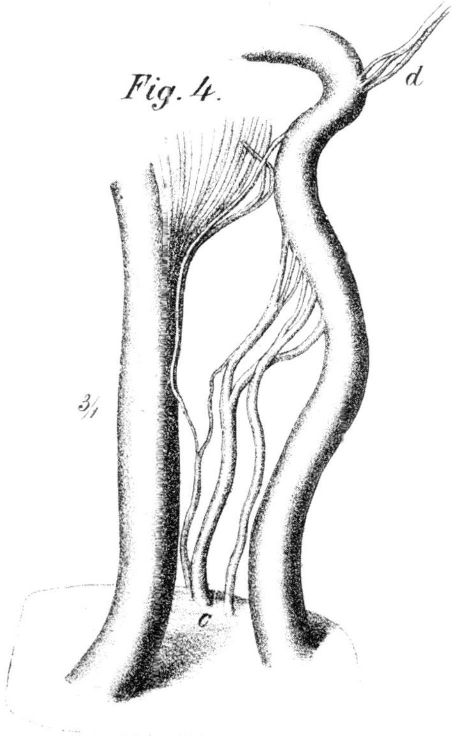

Fig. 4.

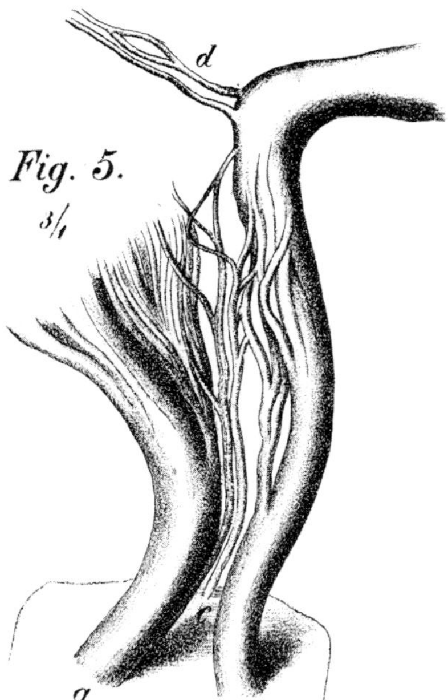

Fig. 5.

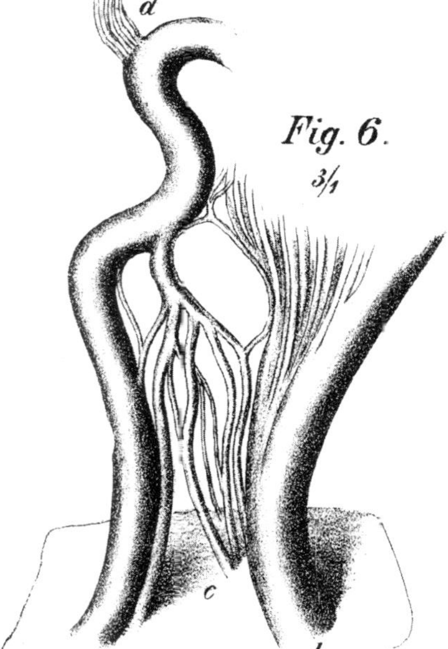

Fig. 6.

Fig. 7.

3/1

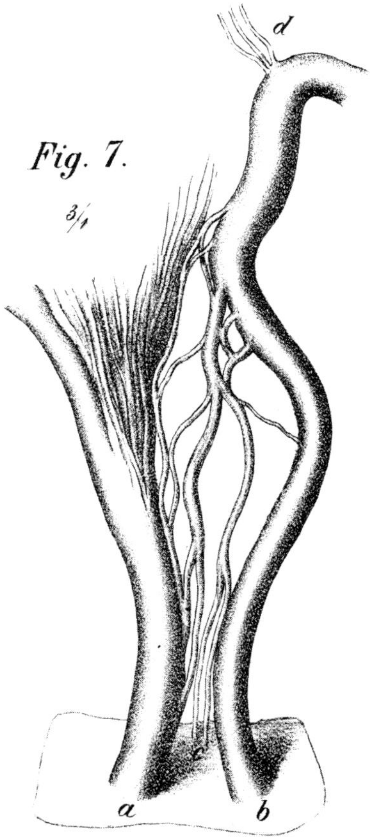

Fig. 8.

3/1

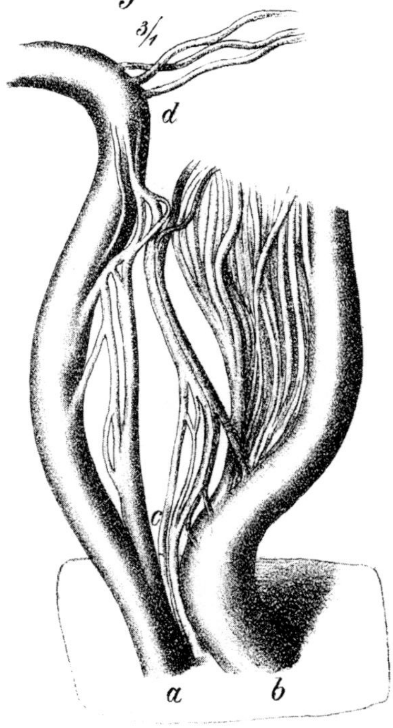

sometimes go from the acoustic to the facial nerve, sometimes vice versa, and sometimes both occur at the same time, when they return to their destination as determined by their origin. Several times I distinctly saw those fibers of the outer anastomosis running toward the genu of the facial nerve; yet I cannot concede that there is a connection with the two petrosal nerves. I shall come back to this later on, when I shall describe the latter and the facial nerve.

II. The Extraocular Motor Nerves

As far as the nerves that move the eyes are concerned—the oculomotor, the trochlear, and the abducens nerves—no anastomoses with other nerves have been mentioned except junctions with the carotid plexus during passage through the outer wall of the cavernous sinus and, as some scientists have said, junctions with the first division of the trigeminal nerve at its passage through the superior orbital fissure.

[Review of the literature, *ed.*]

Among the latter much has been said about an alleged connection between the ophthalmic division of V and the trochlear nerve from which the recurrent nerve or tentorial nerve of the cerebellum originates. This interesting nerve was discovered by Arnold, who at first assumed it to be a branch of the trochlear nerve, although at the place of origin it seemed also connected by a strand with the ophthalmic division [of V—*ed.*]; in addition, it usually has a small ganglion (*De parte ceph. N. sympath.*, p. 19). Later (Kopftheil. *des veg. Nervensyst.*, p. 200, figure VII) [Arnold] believed that it originated from the first division of the trigeminal nerve; he maintained this opinion in his *Anatomie* (Bd. II, p. 830) and in the most recent edition of this (*Tab. Nervor. Cap.*—Tab. III) adding only that a small thread of the carotid nerves joins the fibers of the first division of the trigeminal nerve. Presumably the tentorial nerve runs closely alongside the trochlear nerve and for a time runs within the sheath of that nerve—without, however, forming an anastomosis with it. Longet (*Anat. u. Phys. d. Nervensyst.*, ubers. von Hein, I, p. 151 u. II, p. 335) completely agrees with Arnold, and so does Sappey according to the statement by Cusco (*Anatomie,* II, p. 215). On the other hand, Varrentrapp and Bidder believe that the tentorial nerve has its origin in the trochlear nerve, and they deny that it could originate from the trigeminal nerve. Bidder asserts that he detected a connection between the trochlear nerve and the carotid plexus; for that reason he believed the tentorial nerve to be a sympathetic nerve which runs only for a certain stretch in the same direction as the trochlear nerve (*Neurol. Beobacht.*, p. 11, u. folgol). Krause, too, agrees with this theory (*Anatomie,* II, p. 1128), and he believes that a strand of the carotid plexus at first runs closely alongside the inner aspect of the ophthalmic division, and then of the trochlear nerve, the latter bringing about an apparent connection between those nerves, while it follows the tentorial nerve in a retrograde direction from the trochlear nerve. Finally, Valentin (*Hirn und Nervenlehre,* p. 735) thinks the tentorial nerve is derived from both the ophthalmic division *and* the trochlear nerve, as well as from the carotid plexus, and counts it mainly among the sympathetic nerves.

Results

Examination of the actions of this trochlear nerve requires very great care; I used adults' as well as children's heads and severed the respective nerve portions by dissecting them under the magnifying glass with and without the use of acetic acid. [The results are shown in Figures 9–14.]

(1) It is clear—as described by Arnold and others—that the tentorial nerve is derived from the first branch of the trigeminal nerve, and (2) that it never comes from the trochlear nerve or receives any strands from this source. It must be admitted, however, that a very close and diversified connection exists between the tentorial and the trochlear nerve, for the tentorial lies very close to the trochlear, which at this location is itself not only very close to the ophthalmic division but very often even penetrates the trochlear nerve or surrounds it with two roots; from between these roots the latter [IV nerve—*ed.*] exits. The analysis of the situation can be carried out with sufficient certainty to leave no doubt about the two points mentioned above. On the other hand, I have not succeeded in detecting the third point, namely whether and to what degree the sympathetic nerve is involved in the formation of the tentorial nerve. Between the uppermost edge of the ophthalmic division and the closely adjoining trochlear nerve I find a delicate plexus which seems to be formed chiefly by sympathetic nerves; however, I could not detect with any degree of certainty the relationship of those nerves, or, better, their strands to the tentorial nerve, although several times it looked as if they were involved. In any case this much is certain: the tentorial nerve is a branch of the first division of the trigeminal nerve.

As far as other connections of the three nerves that move the eyes with the first ramus of the trigeminal nerve are concerned, Longet is almost the only one who believes that these connections occur as a rule; he therefore believes that in this manner sensory fibers are carried by those three nerves as a constant component (*Nervensyst.* II, p. 84). Sommering (*Das Sehorgan,* tab. IV, figure 6) shows a picture of a fiber of the nasociliary nerve running toward the uppermost branch of the oculomotor nerve. No other scientist mentions this occurrence concerning the oculomotor nerve, with the exception of Sappey (*Anat.,* II, p. 215), who says that from the uppermost inner edge of the ophthalmic division where the nasociliary nerve begins, it is split into two branches, one of which penetrates into the oculomotor nerve. In regard to the trochlear nerve, the descriptions are more uniform. Sommering was the first to show a picture of its connection with the ophthalmic ramus (*Das Sehorgan,* tab. III, figure V), and almost all the others followed him at least as far as admitting that this connection sometimes exists. On the other hand, Arnold (*Anatomie,* II, p. 880–914) says that in cases where such a connection apparently exists, the ramus that originates from the ophthalmic leaves the trochlear nerve in the orbit and forms a lacrimal branch that seems to start here. Swan, Magendie, Cruveilhier, and others also have made the observation that such a lacrimal branch sometimes proceeds from the trochlear nerve. Longet agrees with Arnold that this branch comes from the ophthalmic, but, as pointed out earlier, he believes that fibers of the latter join the trochlear nerve (Arnold, p. 336). It appears that Sappey (*Anatomie,* II, p. 215) is of the same opinion. Finally, some scientists like Murray and Krause state that a connection occurs occasionally between the trochlear and the infratrochlear nerve by means of a long strand running across the superior oblique muscle.

Findings

I investigated with great care the question of the connection of the first branch of the fifth with the nerves that move the eyes. I separated the portion of the nerve involved with extreme caution, and without the use of acetic acid I examined it under the magnifying glass with a sufficient enlargement. Under the magnifying glass, after the connective tissue has been rendered transparent and the nerves of the eye muscle have been prepared and separated from the first branch of the trigeminal nerve, with which they are closely connected, it is easy to distinguish and follow up each little fiber. In regard to this procedure—used many times—I am in complete accord with Arnold. Never did I see a strand traveling from the trigeminal to the oculomotor and the abducens nerve, and I believe that observations to the contrary are either rare exceptions or are caused by the mistaken belief that the strands of the sympathetic nerve were those of the oculomotor and the abducens nerve. At

FIGURES 9 TO 14

Represent the formation of the tentorial nerve of the cerebellum from the first branch of the trigeminal nerve and its relation to the trochlear nerve. Figures 9, 10, and 12 are taken from children.

C central

P periphery of the nerve in question

a part of the first branch of the trigeminal nerve

b tentorial nerve originating from a portion of the trigeminal nerve pursuing a retrograde course in its relation to the trochlear nerve

c trochlear nerve

e probably sympathetic fibers

f lacrimal accessory nerve

g strands going from the trigeminal to the trochlear nerve

Fig. 9.

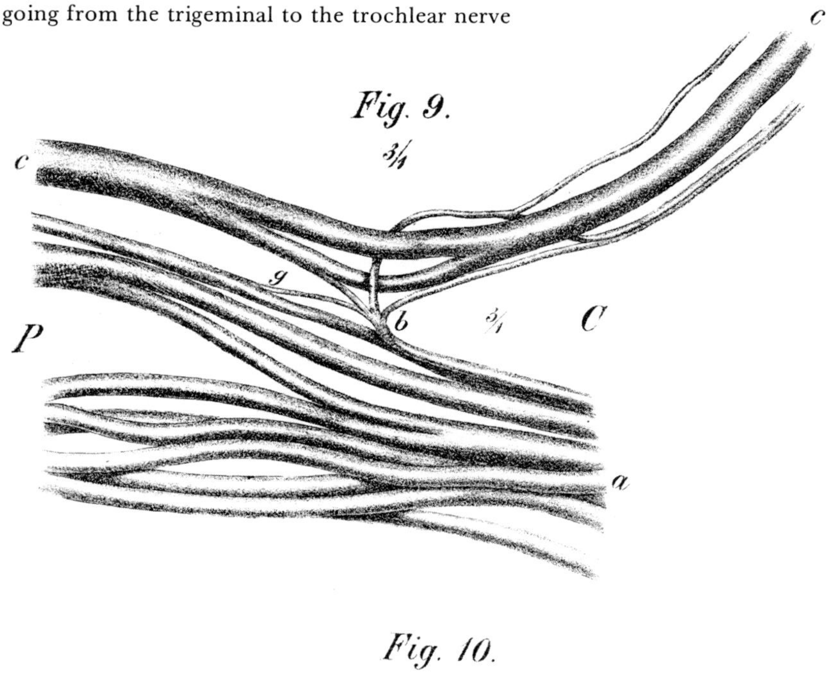

Fig. 10.

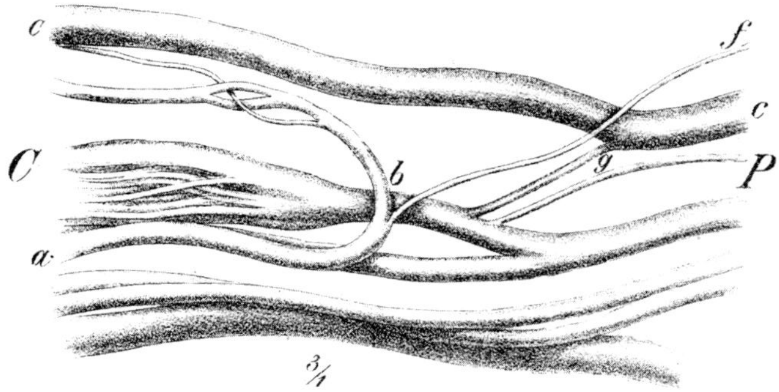

Fig. 11.

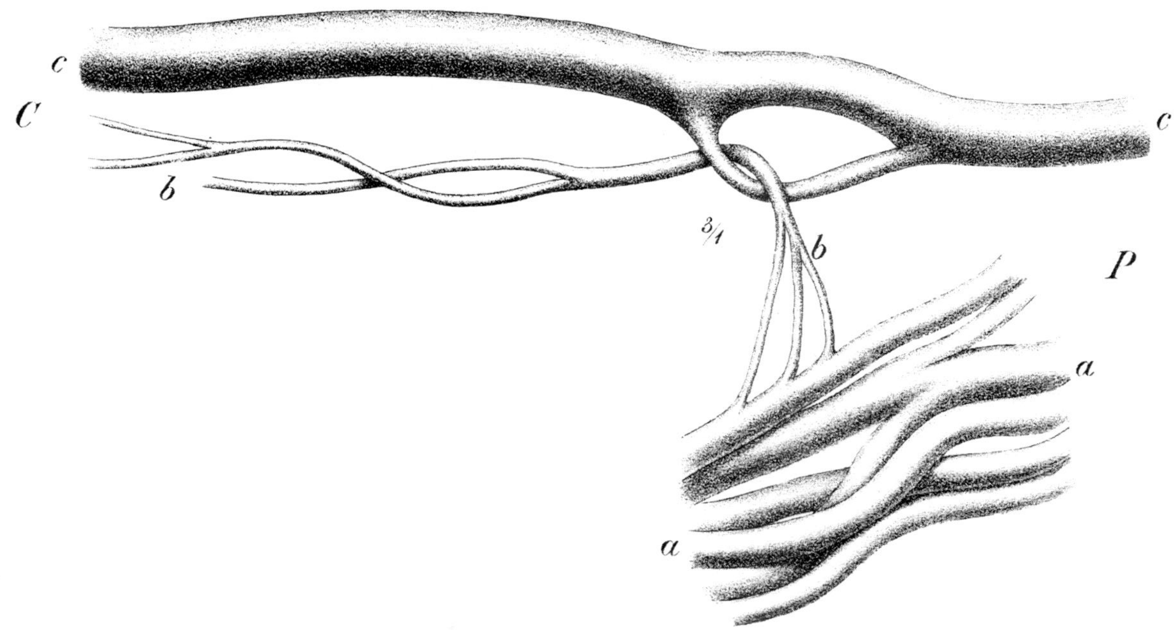

Fig. 12.

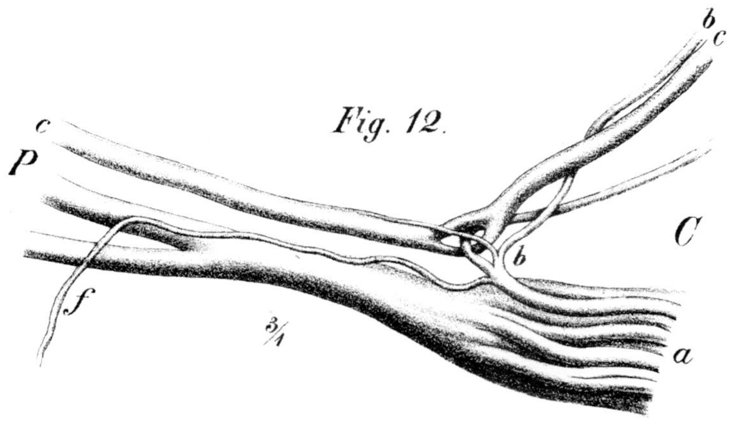

Fig. 13.

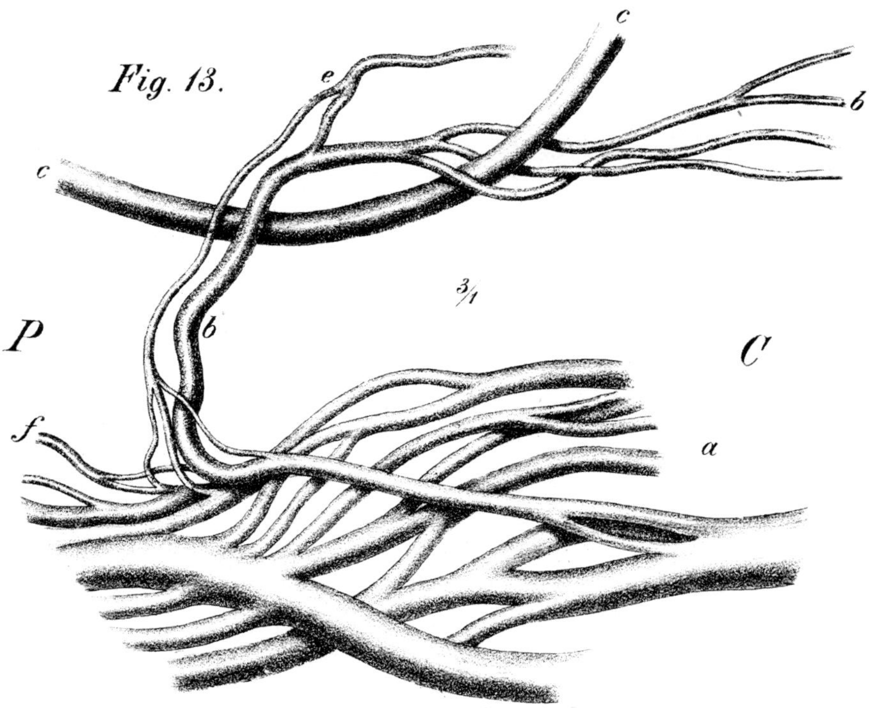

Fig. 14.

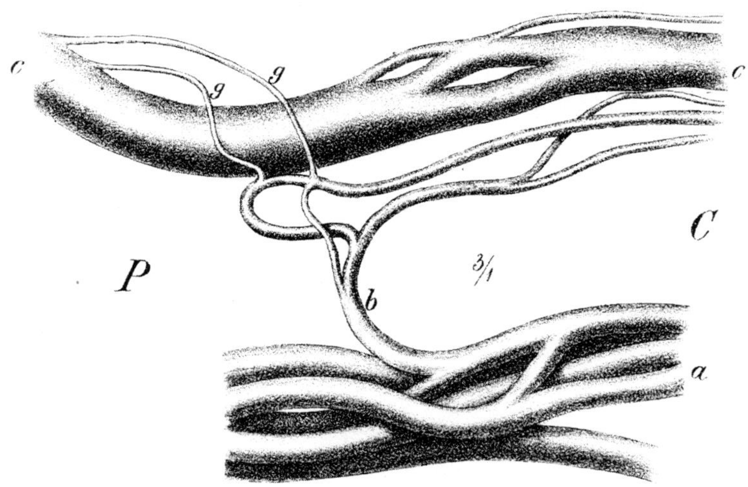

the point where those two nerves pass the internal carotid and the trigeminal nerve, they are surrounded by multitudes of threads of the sympathetic nerves. It can therefore easily happen that a scientist thinks he sees short connecting strands between them and the trigeminal nerve while in reality they belong to the plexus of the sympathetic nerves. The use of acetic acid protects against such an error; it causes the few threads of the sympathetic nerve that are surrounded by strong sheaths to become completely transparent, while the fibers of the trigeminal nerve remain white. In addition, it is not difficult to distinguish the thicker trunks of the nerves moving the eyes, and those of the trigeminal nerve from the finer strands of the sympathetic nerve.

In the case of the trochlear nerve, the situation is different, and here, too, I agree with Arnold. Besides observing the tentorial nerve apparently joining the trochlear, he almost always observes fibers of the first branch of the trigeminal nerve, not only for part of its length running close to the trochlear nerve but also passing into its sheath and, together with the sheath, entering the orbit at the periphery. Usually one can detect that these fibers leave the trochlear nerve in the form of a secondary delicate lacrimal nerve situated alongside the main lacrimal nerve, but I do not venture to decide whether the separation is complete or whether perhaps a few fibers remain inside the trochlear nerve; nor am I certain where they end at the periphery. I believe, however, that the latter is the case, particularly since I saw several times certain fibers passing from the first division* of the trigeminal into the trochlear nerve, after the second lacrimal nerve had already been separated and formed.

Incidentally, this second lacrimal nerve is not always a product of the fibers that have been detached from the trochlear nerve: it often comes directly from the ophthalmic nerve. The reason it is so difficult and often almost impossible to make a definite decision is that the connection between the trochlear and the trigeminal nerve is not formed by one strand alone but by several small strands interwoven in a kind of plexus, in which sympathetic fibers are possibly involved [Figure 15].

*[Confirmed. Ref. *Gray's,* p. 1001, ref. 982. *Ed.*]

FIGURE 15

Apparent anastomosis caused by sympathetic fibers between the trigeminal, oculomotor, and abducens nerves.

a piece of the first branch of the trigeminal nerve

b trochlear nerve

c abducens nerve

d oculomotor nerve

e sympathetic fibers

ff lacrimal nerves I and II from the trigeminal nerve

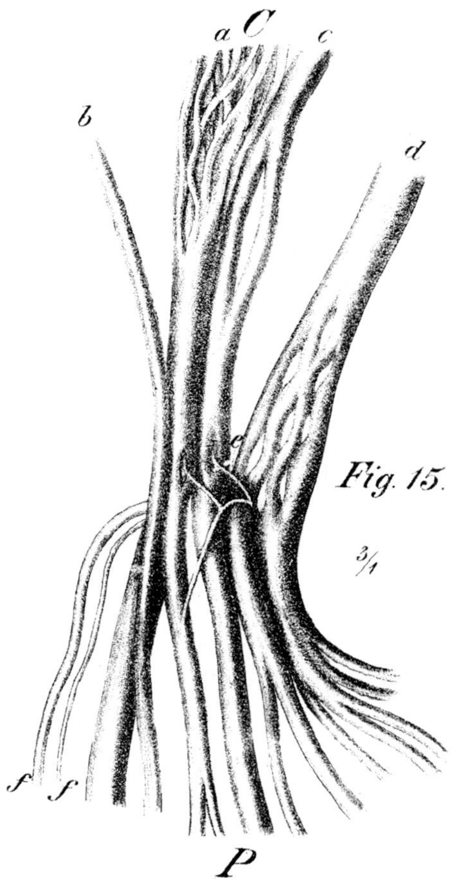

III. The Trigeminal Nerve

In the area of the first division of the trigeminal nerve we first come across the well known anastomosis between the external branch of the lacrimal nerve and the superior ramus of the zygomatico-temporal branch of the second division. Up to the present time no scientist has discussed this anastomosis and whether it carries fibers of the zygomatico-temporal branch to the lacrimal nerve, or vice versa. Sappey (p. 216) states that the connection takes place directly behind the lacrimal gland, and that it forms an arc concave outward. Sommering (*Icon. oculi huma.,* tab. III, figure V) pictures the anastomosis in this shape, although he says, probably in error, that it is a connection with the *third* division of the trigeminal. Usually the shape of the anastomosis is as described above. However, it is not a simple arc in which the fibers run into or lie close to one another; several fine fibers always emerge from the convex side of the arc. These strands penetrate the lacrimal gland where they branch out and sometimes even go to the upper lid. An exact microscopic examination of the slightly compressed nerves shows that those strands are composed of fibers of both nerves in such a way that all of them seem to follow a peripheral course. A few times this did not appear true of all fibers coming together in the anastomosis, but one has to assume that several of them pass from one nerve to the other in the form of a loop, and therefore create a so-called "anastomosis without end." This statement does not imply, however, that I found such a formation, since it is possible that the strands involved separate from one of the two nerves in a retrograde way. Only this much is certain: fibers of the zygomatico-temporal branch from the second branch of the trigeminal nerve branch out at the lacrimal gland [Figures 16-19].

I did not examine the connections of fine terminal branches of the lacrimal nerve with the facial or the superficial temporal nerve [auriculo-temporal—*ed.*] of the third division of the trigeminal nerve, which some authors have mentioned; for they represent in any case only juxtapositions of single fibers of those nerves. [Not so, according to *Gray's. Ed.*]

The supratrochlear nerve originating from the frontal branch of

FIGURES 16 TO 19

The anastomosis between the lacrimal nerve and the zygomatico-temporal:

a zygomatico-temporal

b lacrimal nerve

In Figure 18 the fibers forming anastomoses were pointed into different directions in order to facilitate drawing.

In Figure 19 the *c* represents a branch of the zygomatico-temporal nerve running in a retrograde direction to the orbit.

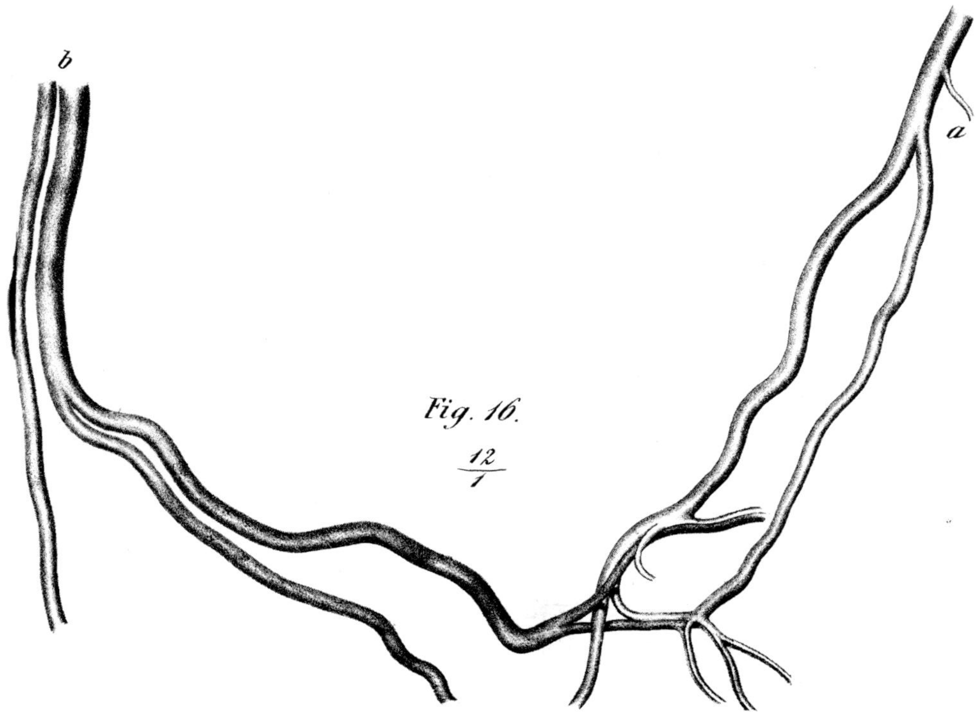

Tab. V.

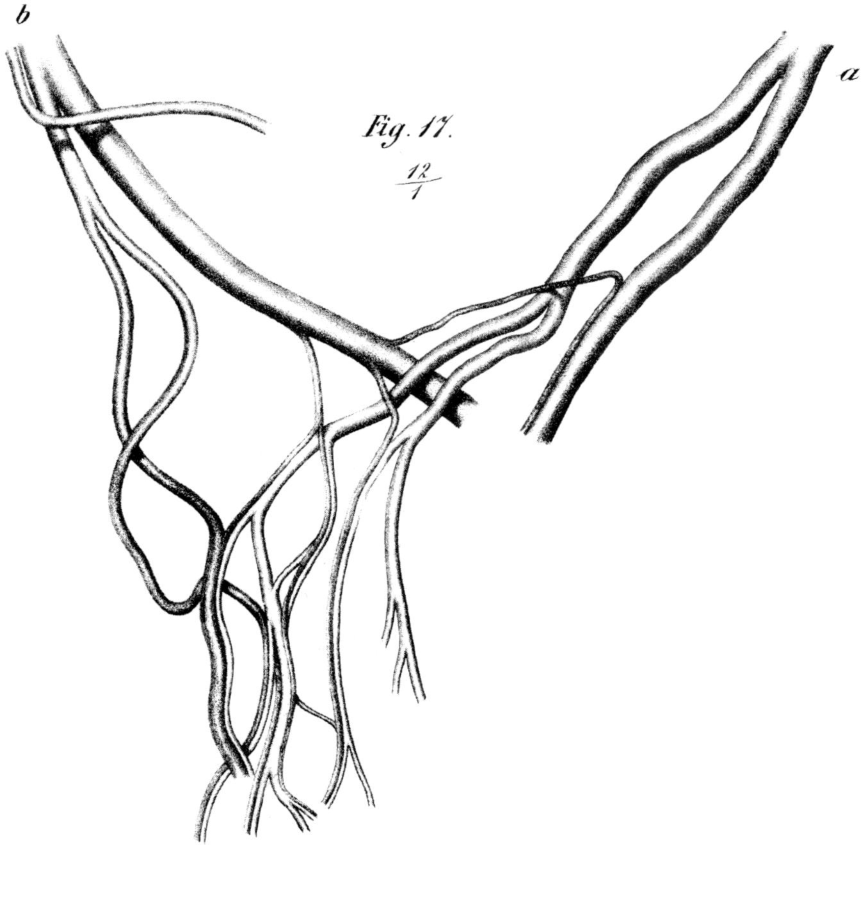

Fig. 18.

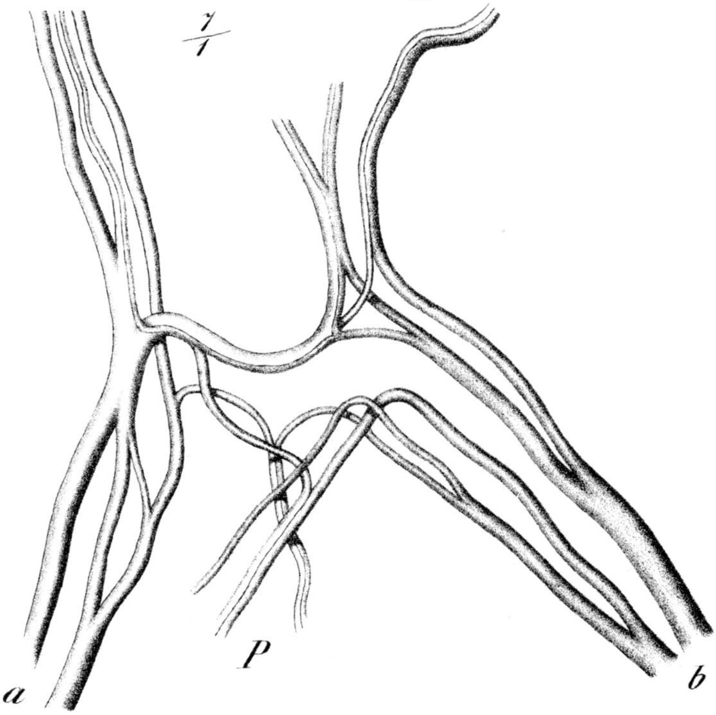

Fig. 19.

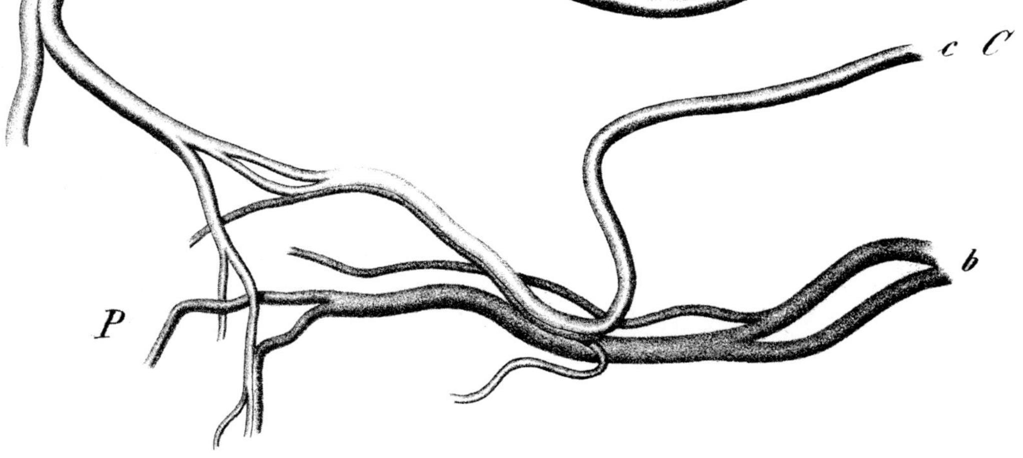

the ophthalmic and the infratrochlear coming from the nasociliary branch of the ophthalmic nerve form an anastomosis very similar to that between the lacrimal nerve and the zygomatico-temporal [Figures 20-23]. I have always seen them, although some scientists say that they appear only once in a while, and not much attention has been paid to them. The anastomosis of the two nerves also forms an arc with its convex side pointing outward, from which a number of small strands leave anteriorly. The microscope shows that those strands come out of fibers of both nerves and that all of them travel in a peripheral course and spread out at the skin and mucous membrane of the inner canthus.

I spent much time and made many preparations of the well known anastomosis between the second branch of the trigeminal nerve (or rather its sphenopalatine ganglion) and the genu of the facial nerve through the so-called vidian nerve [Figures 24-27]. I deem it unnecessary to repeat at this point the often told story of this anastomosis and will confine myself to a review of those opinions prevalent nowadays. It is known and also being taught that this nerve is composed of two strands, one of which, the so-called greater superficial petrosal, connects the spheno-palatine ganglion with the genu of the facial nerve, while the other one, the deep petrosal nerve, connects it with the carotid plexus of the sympathetic nerve. Arnold first described the place where the greater superficial petrosal nerve joins the genu of the facial nerve as a ganglion, and called it the geniculate ganglion. Later he developed the theory that this nerve passes from the facial nerve to the sphenopalatine ganglion and that it acts as its motor root, while the deep petrosal passes from the carotid plexus to the same ganglion and should be regarded as its sympathetic root. Many agreed with this opinion, while others like Meckel had already earlier assumed that the greater superficial petrosal is a branch of the trigeminal going to the facial nerve; Cloquet and Hirzel as well as recent authors like Hyrtl (at least in the earlier editions of his *Anatomie*) claimed that they had followed it across the facial nerve up to the chorda tympani. Finally, there were those who preferred the middle course between these two opinions and declared that the nerve was a composite, running partly from the facial nerve to the sphenopalatine ganglion and partly from the latter to the former. Among those who shared this belief, Beck especially distinguished himself (*Anat. Unter. über das VII und IX Hirnnerven paar*, p. 32), since his statements about the double connection are the most definite ones, and he confirmed them through figures (tab. X, figure 4, and tab. III, figure 6), which did not seem to leave any doubt. In addition, he maintained that he had followed the fibers leaving the facial nerve

FIGURES 20 TO 23

Anastomosis between the superior and the inferior trochlear nerve.

a superior trochlear nerve

b inferior trochlear nerve

Figure 20 looks as if it contains a nerve loop without end; therefore, it may be decided arbitrarily whether it goes from the inferior to the superior trochlear nerve, or vice versa.

Fig. 20.

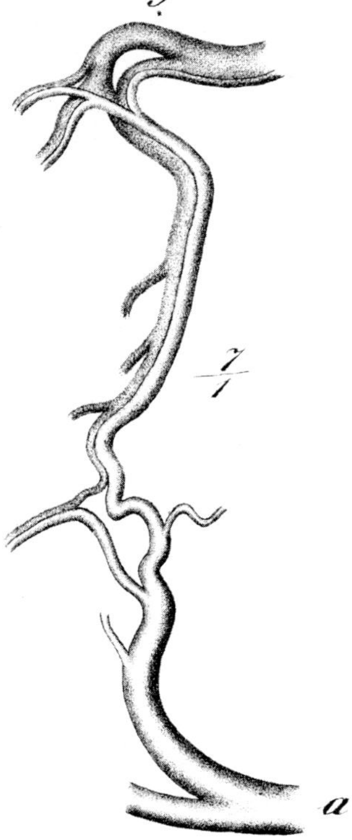

Fig. 21.

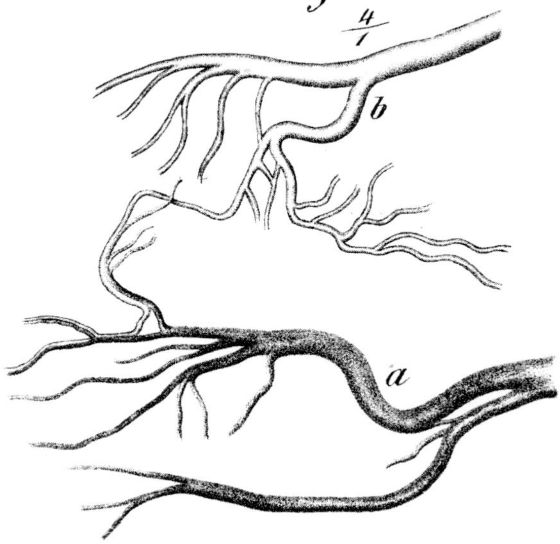

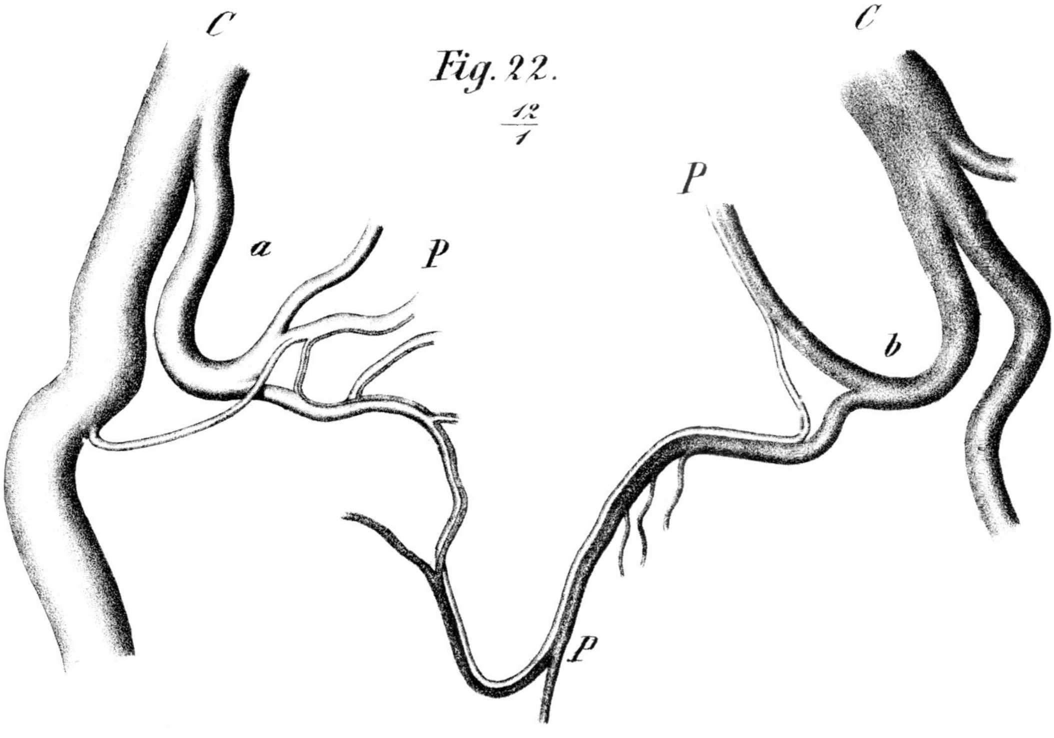
C
Fig. 22.
12/1
C
P
a
P
b
P

Fig. 23.

$\frac{12}{1}$

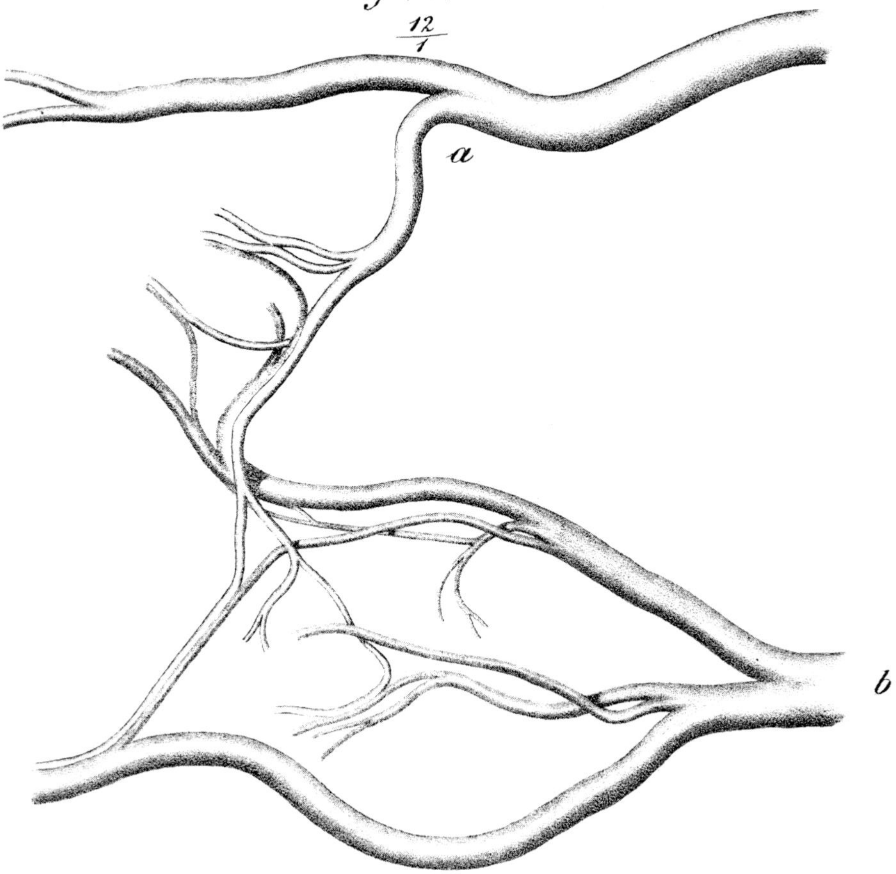

through the sphenopalatine ganglion up to the posterior palatine nerves; he also felt sure he had seen that the fibers going from this ganglion to the facial nerve do not pass into any branch of this nerve during its passage through the Fallopian canal, but that together with it they come out through the stylomastoid foramen at the outer edge of this nerve.

I dealt repeatedly with the questions above and made many relevant preparations from adults' and children's heads on fresh nerves, and on those treated with acetic acid under the magnifying glass with pins, and with pressure using the compressor. The following are the results of these experiments: they do not compare favorably with the theories.

In its first part going through the vidian [pterygoid] canal up to the exit of the deep petrosal, as well as in its second part, as the greater superficial petrosal up to the genu of the facial nerve—the vidian nerve is by no means a single strand, nor does it consist of two strands, but at all points it is a plexus which in its first part is represented by a composite of the strands of the greater superficial petrosal and the deep petrosal and in its second part by a separation and reunion of the strands of the latter. I was able to convince myself of the reality of these findings through slightly compressed preparations that were made clearer by means of acetic acid.

As far as the deep petrosal nerve is concerned, I agree completely with those who say that it is a sympathetic nerve which passes from the carotid plexus to the sphenopalatine ganglion. This cannot, however, be concluded from the direction of its course and its manner of joining with its two terminal points. This would allow the assumption that it exits from the ganglion and passes to the sympathetic nerve as well as vice versa. The microscopic examination of the situation of the fibers of this deep petrosal nerve characterizes it completely as a sympathetic nerve consisting of fine nerves surrounded by a strong sheath, while those of the greater superficial petrosal are much thicker and resemble the other cranial nerves.

On the other hand, I have remained completely in the dark about the origin of this greater superficial petrosal nerve, inasmuch as I cannot state that it originates either from fibers of the trigeminal nerve or from the facial nerve; indeed it is merely a connection between the sphenopalatine and the geniculate ganglion. I never succeeded—in contrast to Beck's contention—in following its fibers through the sphenopalatine ganglion to any other nerves, since I always lost them in these ganglia before I had a chance (with my method of experiments and before I had made a sufficient attempt) to find out whether they join with these ganglionic masses [Figures 28-30]. The same fact applies to the connection with the genicu-

FIGURES 24 TO 27

The vidian nerve, or the anastomosis between the sphenopalatine ganglion and the geniculate ganglion.

Figures 24 and 27 show only the plexus between the greater superficial and the deep petrosal in connection with the sphenopalatine ganglion.

a sphenopalatine ganglion

b geniculate ganglion

c carotid nerve

d greater superficial petrosal nerve

e greater deep petrosal nerve

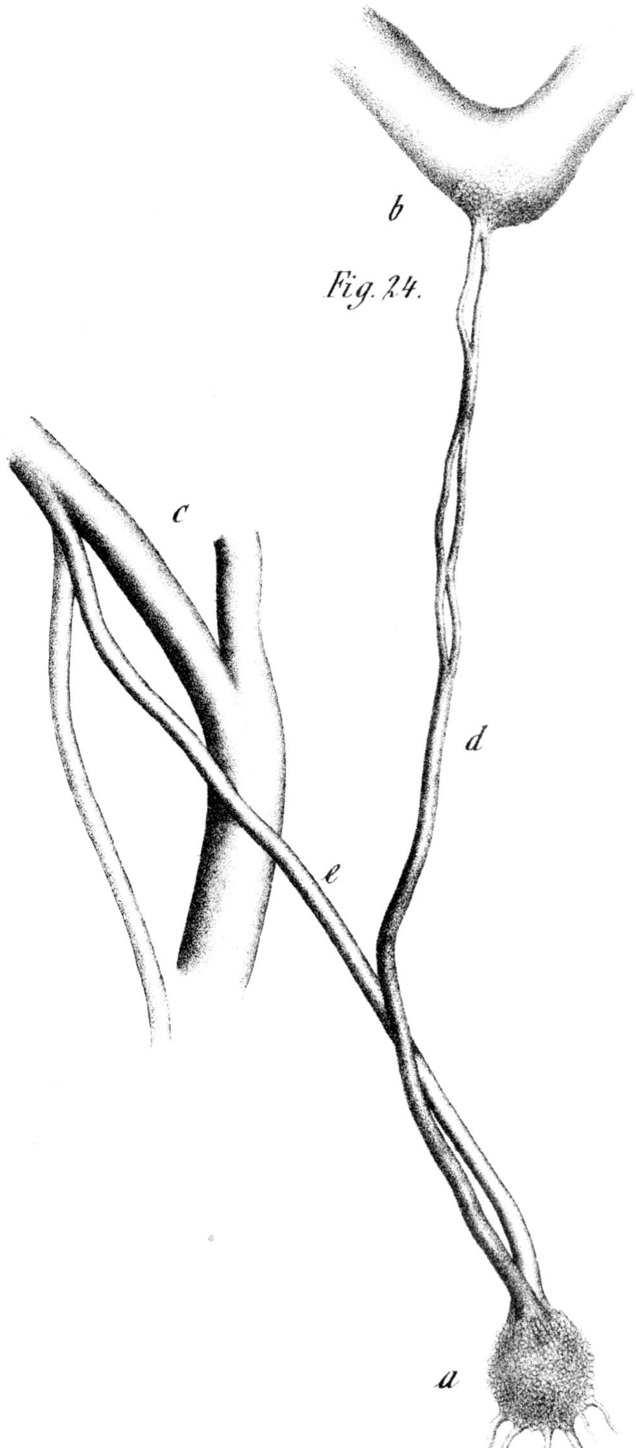

Fig. 24.

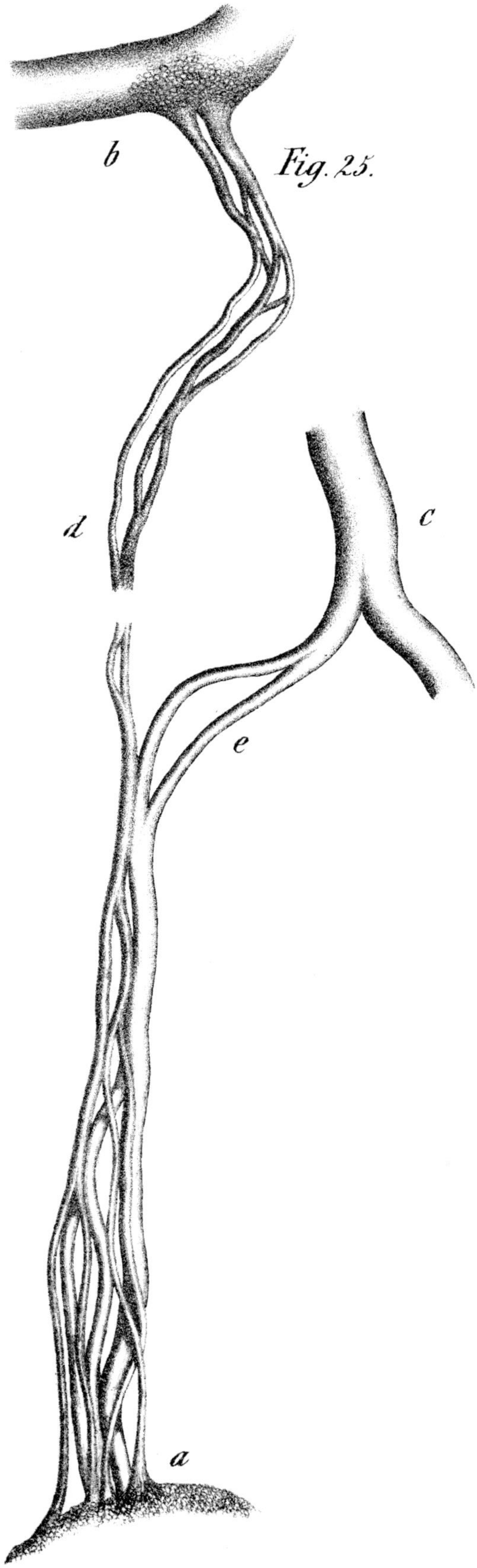

Fig. 25.

Fig. 26.

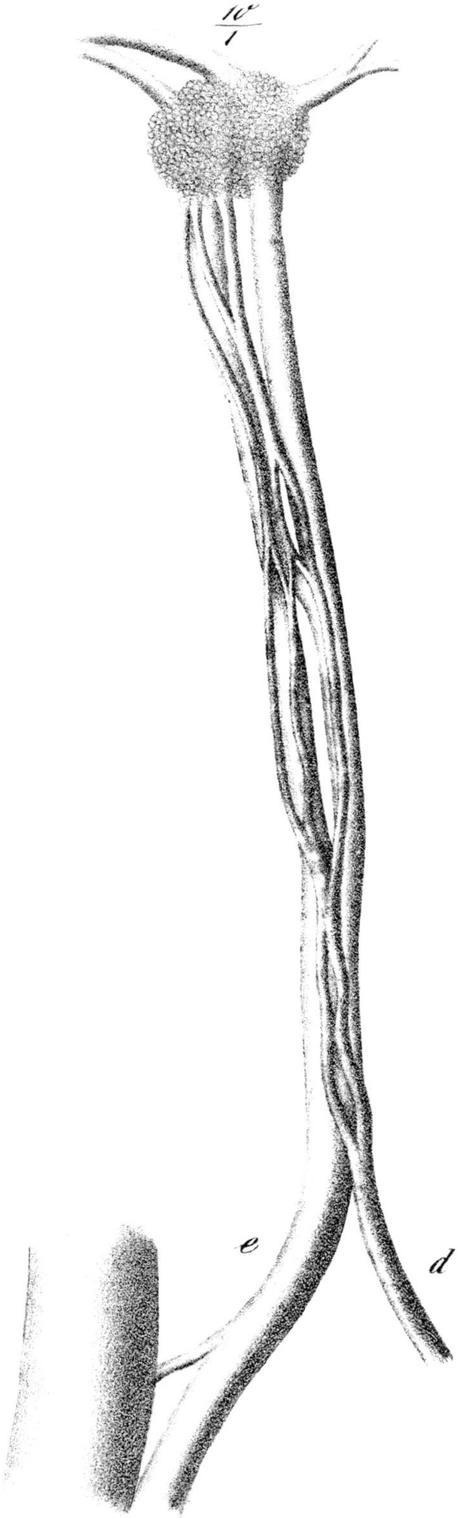

Fig. 27.

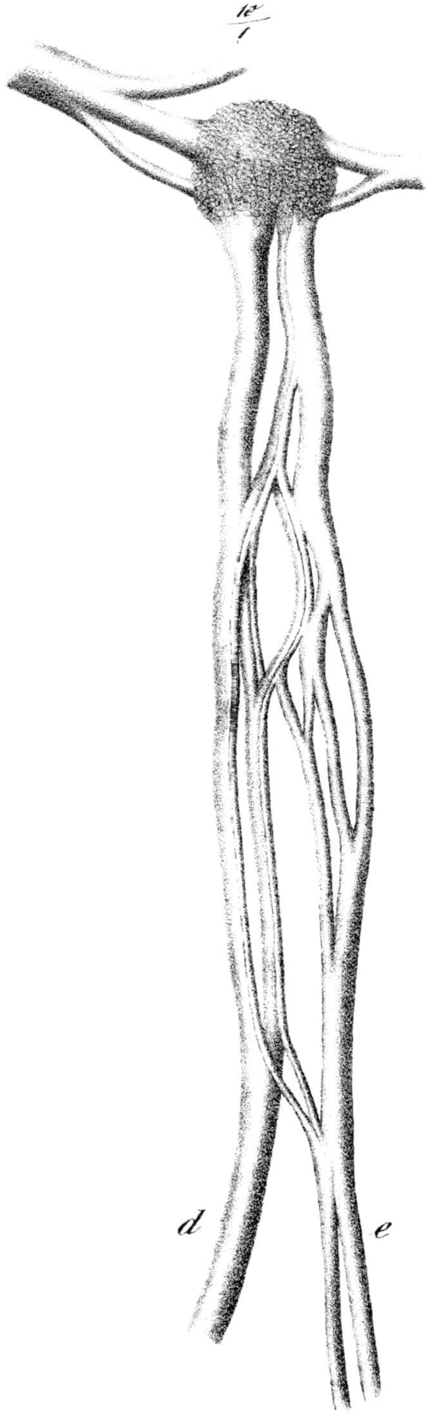

FIGURES 28 TO 30

These show the sphenopalatine ganglion and its connection with the vidian nerve which cannot be traced through the ganglion to a branch of the sphenopalatine nerve, because it is interrupted by the ganglia.

a superior maxillary ramus of the trigeminal nerve

b sphenopalatine nerve

c sphenopalatine ganglion

d vidian nerve

[Note error in numbering two Figures 29. The bottom one should be Figure 30. *Ed.*]

Fig. 28.

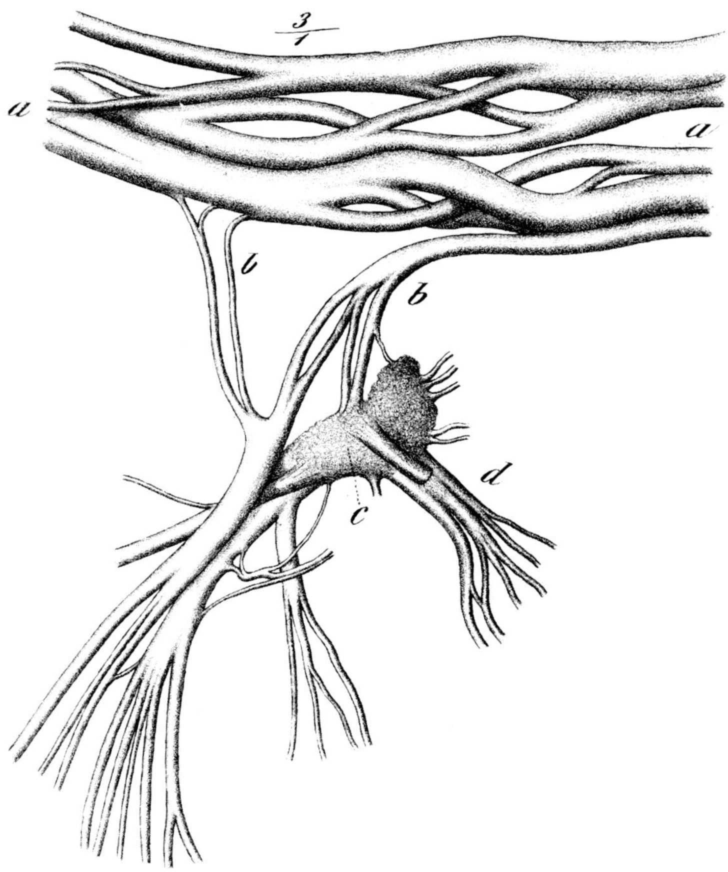

Fig. 29.

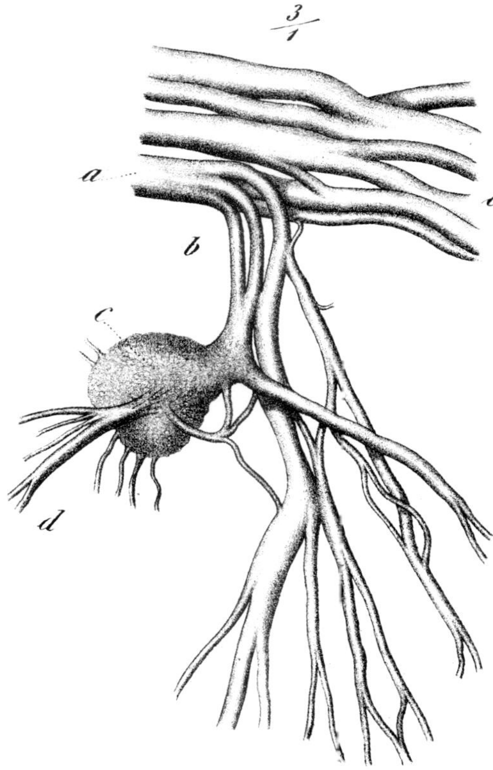

Fig. 29.

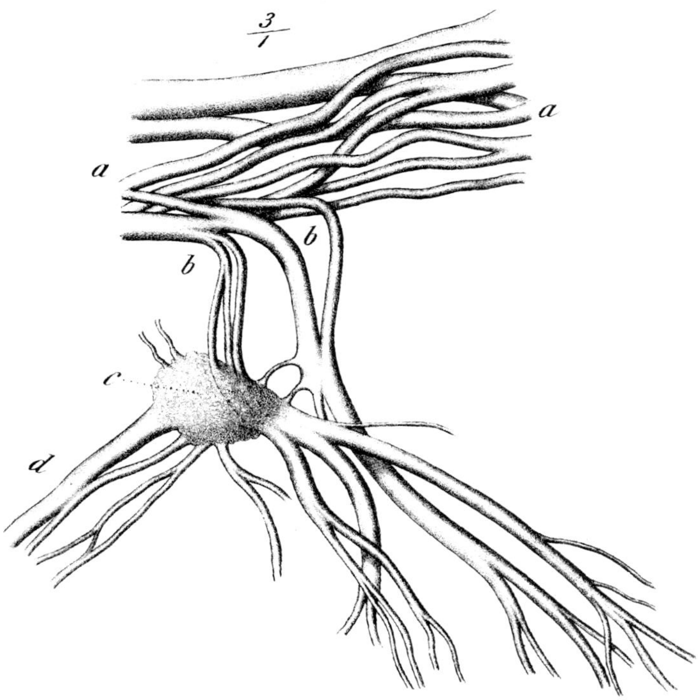

late ganglion. The greater superficial petrosal always joins the latter through at least two and often three fibers situated closely together, which during their course toward the sphenopalatine ganglion get together in a plexiform manner. I believe it is impossible to follow within the geniculate ganglion the continuation of the fibers that branch out in the ganglion. It cannot be done toward the central end of the facial nerve or toward its periphery, and I am forced to believe that Beck's pictures are erroneous, although I admit that the solution of the problem is very difficult, since one has to deal with a nerve as thick as the facial nerve is at this spot. Nevertheless, after having made a great many experiments with preparations derived from adults and children, with and without the sheaths treated with acetic acid, dissected with a pin, and pressed with the compressor, I must insist that my conclusion is correct. I see only one explanation for the error committed by Hirzel and Cloquet, as well as by Beck, in regard to a peripheral course within the facial nerve by the entire petrosal or by a part of its fibers: If pressure is used on a facial nerve deprived of its sheath, a group of fibers is sometimes separated on the outer side of the genu, and this group could be regarded mistakenly as a connection with the fibers of the petrosal which enter the genu. The most meticulous study of just those cases, however, has convinced me that this can only happen in a person's imagination. As mentioned above in regard to the auditory nerve, Arnold and Valentin have stated that it is possible to follow the fibers of the outer anastomosis of the auditory nerve with the facial nerve up to the greater superficial petrosal. But even if this is sometimes possible up to the genu of the facial nerve, I cannot but agree with Sappey, who derives these fibers from Wrisberg's nervus intermedius and says that at this point they disperse and that there is no proof of a direct connection with the fibers of the greater superficial petrosal. I repeat that the fibers of the petrosal disappear into ganglia which can be distinctly recognized even with a rather slight enlargement and often are slightly pigmented; here, too, I leave the question open as to whether they are joined.

It follows that the greater superficial petrosal is only a connection between the two ganglia. I cannot say whether or in what manner its fibers are connected by means of the ganglion with the facial or the trigeminal nerve or with both.

It will be best to discuss the anastomoses of the third branch of the trigeminal nerve with the facial, the glossopharyngeal, and the hypoglossal nerve when I come to the discussion of those nerves.

IV. The Facial Nerve

The facial nerve is one of the cranial nerves which during its course forms the greatest number of so-called anastomoses. I have already mentioned above an apparent connection with the acoustic nerve in the internal auditory meatus and have shown that in fact it is only an apparent one brought about through a few small fibers of Wrisberg's nervus intermedius which belongs to it. I have also talked in detail about the connection of the genu of the facial nerve with the second branch of the trigeminal nerve and pointed out that the greater superficial petrosal is a connection between the geniculate ganglion of the facial nerve and the sphenopalatine ganglion, and that the nerve passes into this ganglion. In the same manner I shall demonstrate that the apparent anastomosis between the genu of the facial nerve and the tympanic plexus, or rather the lesser superficial petrosal nerve, is in fact not an anastomosis but only a connection with a small vessel branch. I shall discuss this when I come to the glossopharyngeal nerve.

When we continue to follow the course of the facial nerve through the Fallopian canal, we find the next connection with another nerve to be the well known one with the lingual nerve of the third branch of the trigeminal nerve through the chorda tympani. Because of its strange course this nerve has been studied for a long time, and quite a few detailed descriptions have been published. I feel justified, therefore, to assume that its history is generally known. It has been generally agreed upon that the chorda tympani is a branch of the facial nerve which, after having made its way through the cavity runs close to the lingual nerve, partially running peripherally inside the latter and partially entering the lingual nerve; Arnold called it the motor root of the latter. Cloquet, Ribes, Hirzel, Hyrtl, and others maintain that the chorda originates from the superficial petrosal, while others, mainly Arnold and Beck—as said before—rightly oppose that theory. Beck and Valentin say that they have followed the chorda tympani upward in the trunk of the facial nerve to its roots (p. 48) and Cusco even believes that it comes from Wrisberg's nervus intermedius [the taste fibers of course do. *Ed.*] (Sappey, p. 258). Only Valentin (p. 447) and Longet (p. 359) are of the opinion that when the chorda tympani leaves the facial nerve, it not only consists of fibers originating from the center of the latter, but also gives up some fibers running peripherally into the facial nerve. Valentin does not say whence these fibers supposedly come. According to Longet they originate from the lingual nerve, and he therefore calls the chorda tympani a mixed nerve.

I have frequently and meticulously studied the location where the chorda tympani leaves the facial nerve, a rather difficult task because of the thickness of the facial nerve [Figures 31-40].

The trunk of the nerve must be placed in such a way that the chorda tympani points away from its edge. After its sheath has been rendered brighter with acetic acid, or, even better, cautiously stripped off—having become contracted and gelatinized by means of acetic acid, the nerve must be compressed—the following can be observed: (1) the majority of its fibers come from the trunk of the facial nerve; (2) it would be an impossible undertaking to follow isolated fibers upward in the trunk of the facial nerve possibly to the greater superficial petrosal or to the roots of the facial nerve, because, as Sappey rightly states, during their course the portions of the facial nerve become intertwined like a net; (3) in many if not all cases, a small part of the fibers of the chorda tympani turn at their starting point peripherally toward the trunk of the facial nerve and merge with it. I am not able to say where they go, but what I have stated is a definite fact. In addition, I would like to mention here that in many cases I distinctly saw close to the origin a very thin, small strand leaving the central end of the chorda tympani. As far as I know, no one has ever mentioned this. I cannot describe, however, its peripheral course, because it is much too fine to be followed. [He was correct. A connection does go to the otic ganglion. *Ed.*]

In regard to the question of the point of origin of the fibers that pass peripherally from the chorda tympani into the facial nerve, it is necessary to begin by examining their course and then their connection with the lingual nerve. As to the former, several anatomists —Caldani, Langenbeck, Bock, Hirzel, Valentin—have claimed that they saw small strands going from the chorda tympani toward the tensor tympani during passage through the tympanic cavity as well as after leaving it. Like others, I have not been able to detect anything similar. But as far as I know, first Krause (*Anatomie,* II, p. 1135) and later Valentin (p. 446), Cusco, Hirschfeld, and Sappey (p. 258) did sometimes see a small strand from the otic ganglion merging with the chorda. These could possibly enter the chorda tympani centrally and then pass peripherally into the facial nerve, and may originate from the otic ganglion or from the third ramus of the trigeminal nerve. [They originate from both. *Ed.*]

FIGURES 31 TO 40

The figures show the relations of the chorda tympani.

a facial nerve

b chorda tympani

c nerve strand as it often originates close to b

d otic ganglion

e connecting strands between the otic ganglion and the chorda tympani

[Bischoff omitted "f" in his legends and in his figures. *Ed.*]

g connecting strands between the lingual nerve and the chorda tympani

h lingual nerve

i lingual ganglion

k auricular branch of the vagus

Figures 31 and 32 show how all fibers of the chorda tympani leave the facial nerve centrally.

Figure 33 shows that although the major part of the fibers of the chorda tympani come from the facial nerve centrally, a small portion enters the facial nerve peripherally.

Figures 34 and 35 show portions of the chorda tympani entering the facial nerve peripherally, even running separately from the trunk.

Figure 36 shows the connecting strand between the otic ganglion (d) and a branch of the lingual nerve (g) with the chorda tympani (b). Some of the former enter the chorda centrally and may be fibers that in Figures 32–35 run peripherally from the chorda into the facial nerve.

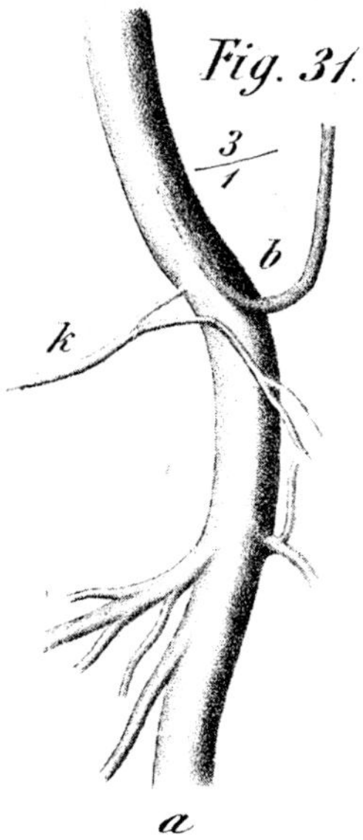

Fig. 31.

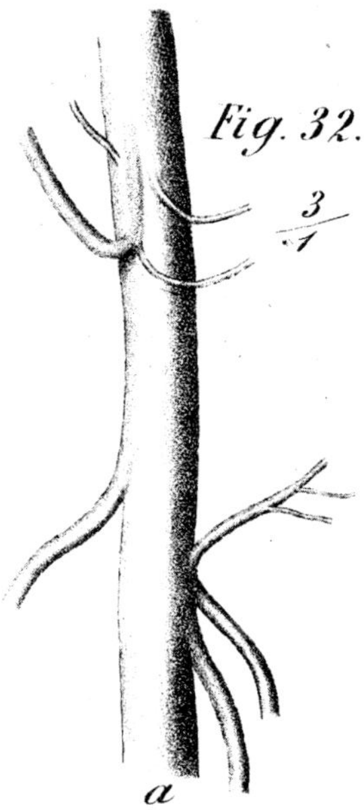

Fig. 32.

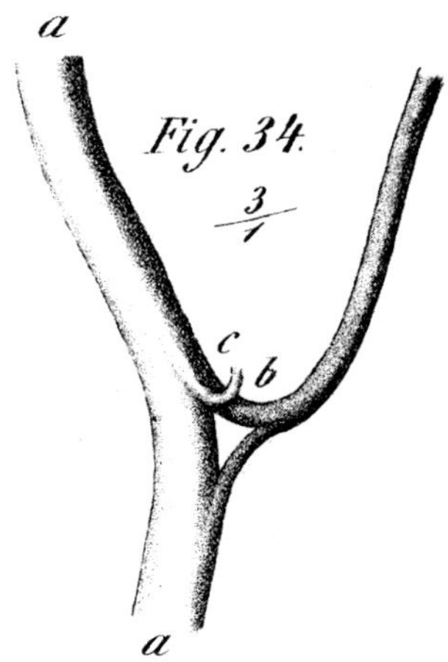

Fig. 34.

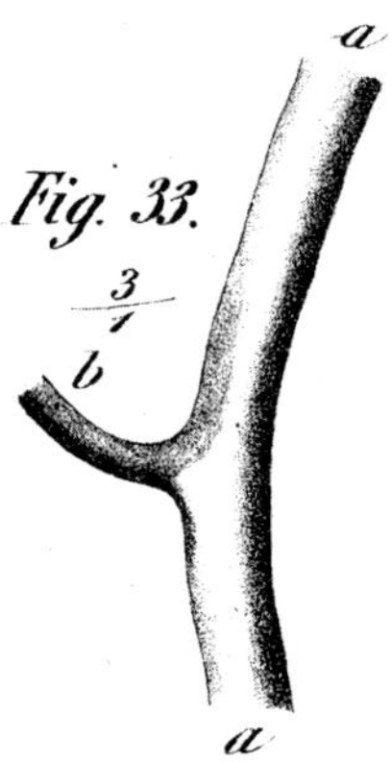

Fig. 33.

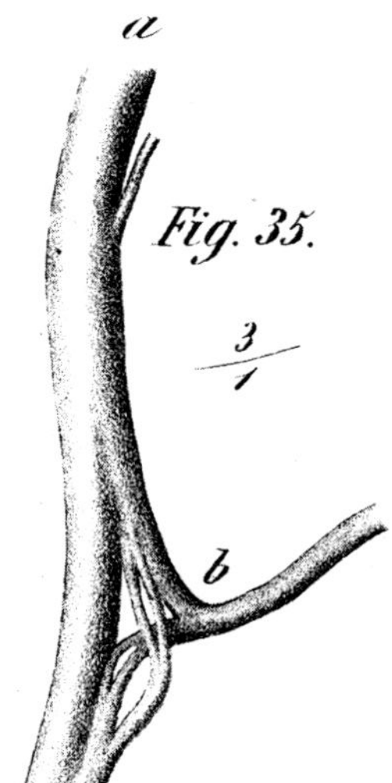

Fig. 35.

Fig. 36.

$\frac{6}{1}$

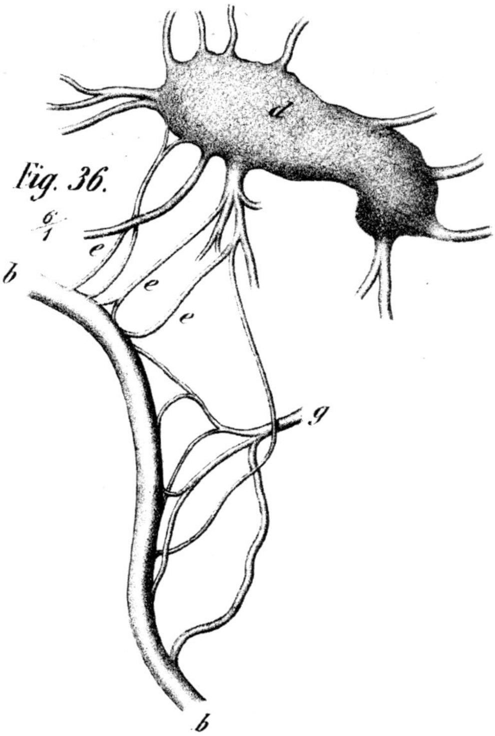

Fig. 37.

$\frac{6}{1}$

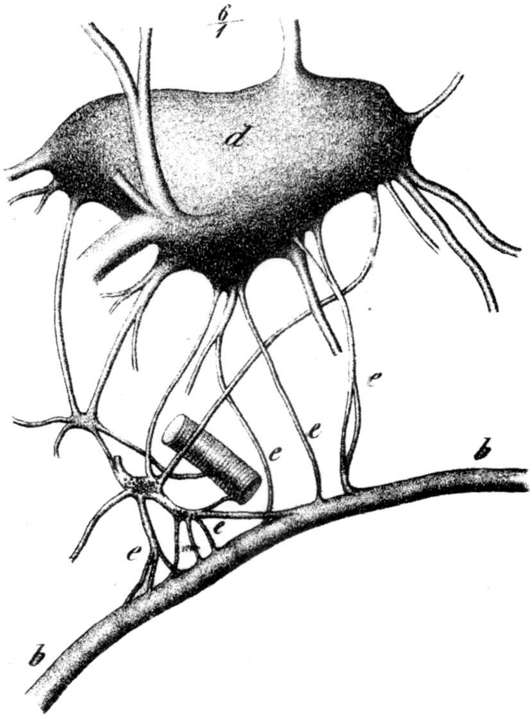

Fig. 38. 6/1

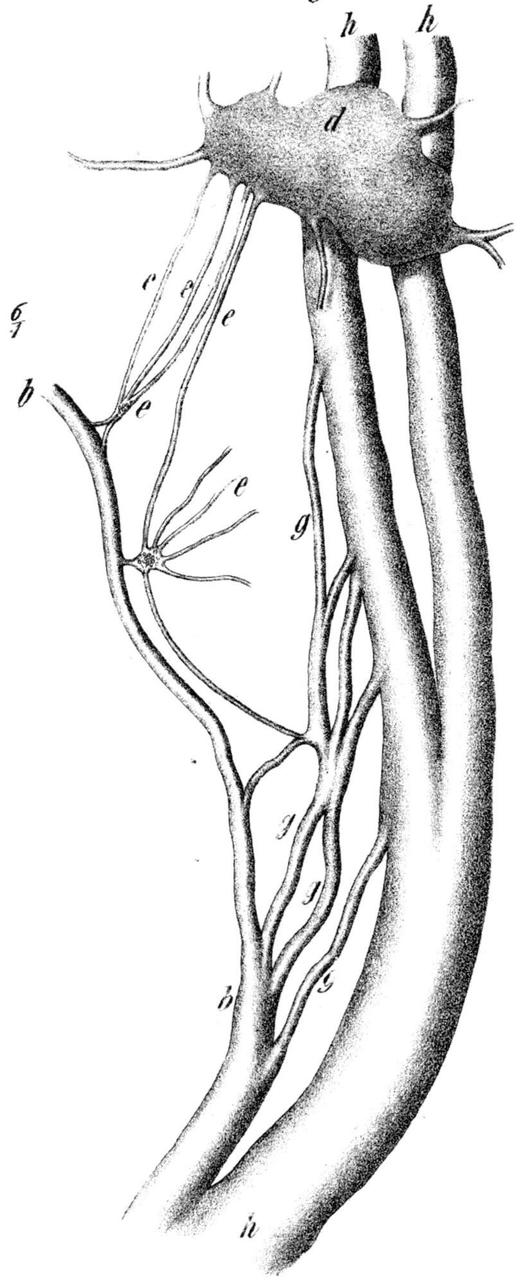

Fig. 39.

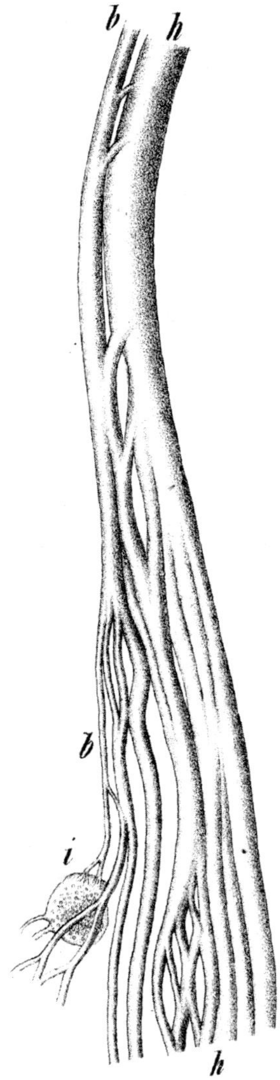

Fig. 40. $\frac{6}{1}$

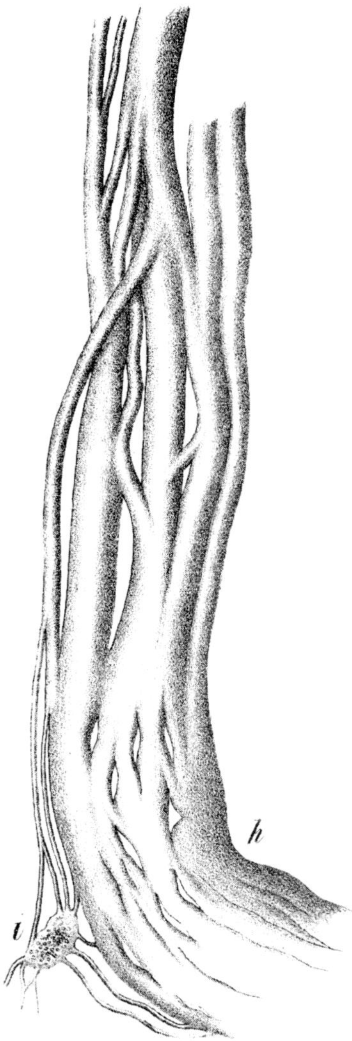

The study of this question presents great difficulties, since the small strands coming from the otic ganglion are extremely fragile and to examine the ganglion and its surrounding area is therefore a complicated procedure. But I always saw several ganglionic fibers entering the chorda, and among them certain ones entered in the direction of the trunk; they may run toward the facial nerve and peripherally pass into it. These connecting strands between the otic ganglion and the chorda tympani usually form a small plexus interspersed with the ganglion. But the same cannot be said of the ganglion. Because of the reciprocal connection of this nerve with the chorda tympani, the exchange of fibers occurs only in a peripheral direction. However, together with Sappey, I must object to the usual opinion that the fibers of the chorda tympani can be followed all the way to the lingual [submandibular–*ed.*] ganglion. During their further course the portions of the facial nerve form such a complicated netlike plexus that I believe this opinion to be unjustified as far as their anatomy is concerned, although there may be facts physiologically pointing to the possibility that the chorda tympani participates in the lingual [submandibular–*ed.*] ganglion and the nerves leaving it.

I now come to an anastomosis of the facial nerve with the auricular branch of the vagus, whose discoverer (Arnold) has been greatly doubted in the past [Figures 41-50]. According to Arnold, who was the first to give a detailed description of the latter nerve, it originates from the jugular ganglion of the vagus nerve as well as a thin root from the glossopharyngeal nerve; it runs across the jugular fossa and through an opening at the back wall of this fossa into the Fallopian canal; here it crosses the facial nerve, joins the latter by means of an ascending and descending branch, and goes into the mastoid canaliculus, where it splits into two branches, one of which joins the deep auricular ramus of the facial nerve while the other branches out in the skin behind the ear. To this connection of the auricular nerve of the vagus with the facial nerve Arnold ascribes the sensory function of the latter (which has already been noticed) when it leaves the mastoid foramen. Arnold does not express an opinion about the question where the branch that descends from the facial nerve and joins the auricular nerve may go, nor does he say in what direction this connection occurs.

Most of his successors have agreed with Arnold's findings. But Beck denies the existence of the passage of fibers of the auricular [branch of the vagus] to the facial nerve and maintains that both connecting small strands go from the facial to the auricular nerve (p. 50). Arnold declares this apodictic assumption to be worthless and he appears to be right, inasmuch as Beck does not say in what direction those fibers of the facial nerve go after they have joined

FIGURES 41 TO 50

The relations of the auricular branch of the vagus:

a facial nerve

b vagus

c glossopharyngeal nerve

d auricular branch of the vagus

e its origin from the glossopharyngeal nerve

f its origin from the vagus

g its roots running peripherally in the vagus or the glossopharyngeal

h fibers of the facial nerve passing centrally from the facial into the auricular nerve

i trunk of the auricular crossing over the facial nerve

k portion of the auricular nerve passing peripherally into the facial nerve

l chorda tympani

m tympanic branch of the glossopharyngeal nerve

Figure 41 shows the entire course of the auricular branch of the vagus. Here it is almost totally derived from the glossopharyngeal with its fibers (3) ascending along its trunk, which seem to run toward its rootlets. However, a certain portion of the fibers (g) also turns peripherally into the trunk of the glossopharyngeal nerve. At the facial nerve it is divided into four branches. Two (i.i.) pass above it, one (h) comes centrally from the facial nerve and probably merges (g) with the glossopharyngeal, while a very small one (h) enters the facial nerve peripherally.

Figure 42 also shows the entire course of the auricular nerve. Here one of its roots (g) turns around peripherally at the vagus; this root probably originates from the strand that leaves the facial nerve peripherally (h). The two strands (i.i.) pass peripherally across the facial nerve. The trunk was composed of two strands.

Figures 44, 45, and 46 show separately the origin of the auricular nerve from the vagus and from the glossopharyngeal nerve. Figure 44 shows a root (g) passing peripherally into the vagus.

Figures 47 and 48 show separately and exactly the origin of the auricular from the vagus and from the glossopharyngeal nerve (a) from outside and (b) from inside. There are two small strands entering the vagus peripherally, but the auricular nerve is also composed of two strands.

Figure 49. The trunk (i) of the auricular nerve which crosses over the facial nerve is reversed, so that the connections with the facial nerve may be better visible; one of them (h) goes to the auricular and the other one (k) turns peripherally with two fibers from the auricular into the facial nerve.

Figure 50 shows a case where the auricular (k) merged completely with the facial nerve. Here the sheath of the facial nerve was pulled off to make sure that the facts were correct. But one small thread (h) also came from the facial nerve and went peripherally into the auricular, and they were joined by still another small strand (x) whose origin is unknown to me.

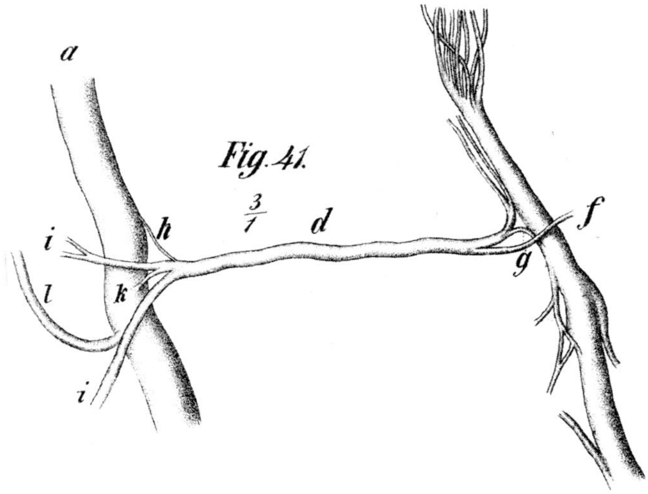

Fig. 41. 3/1

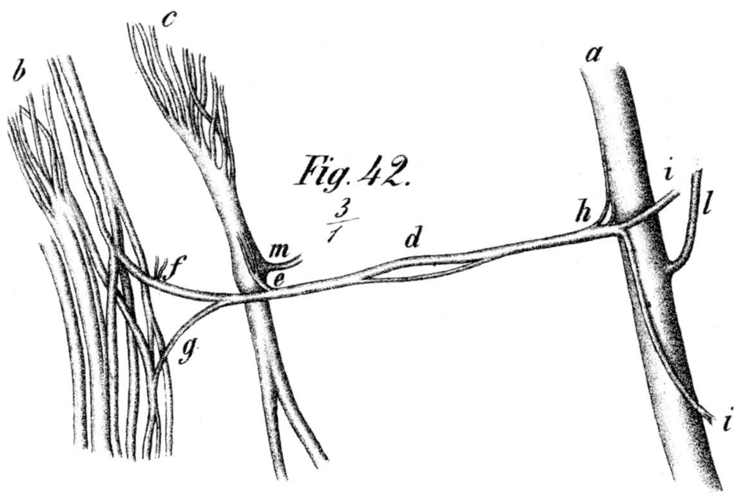

Fig. 42. 3/1

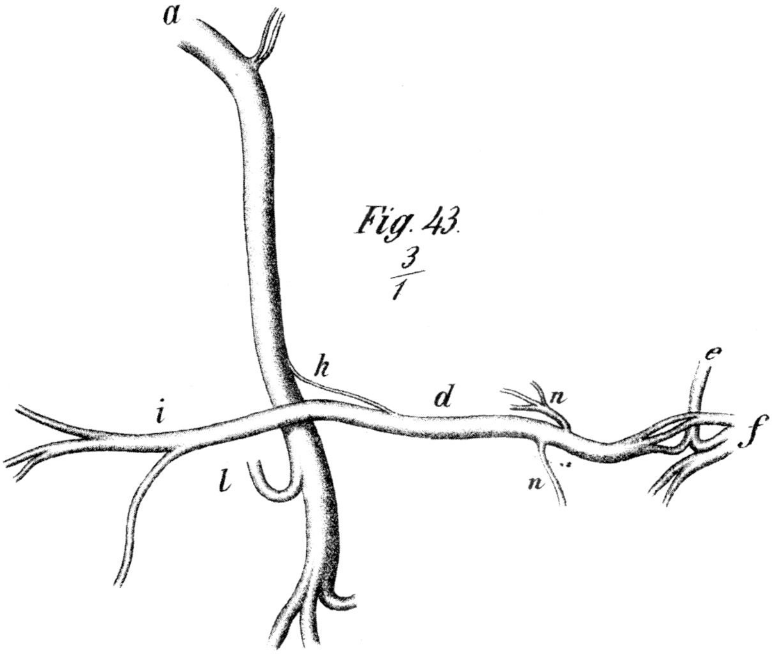

Fig. 43.
$\frac{3}{1}$

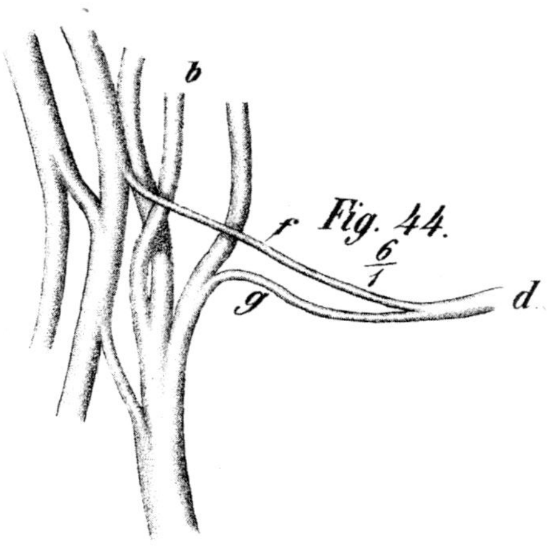

Fig. 44.
$\frac{6}{1}$

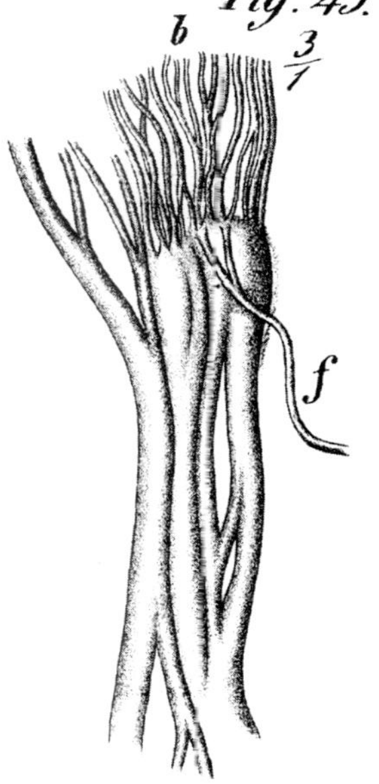

Fig. 45.
$\frac{3}{1}$

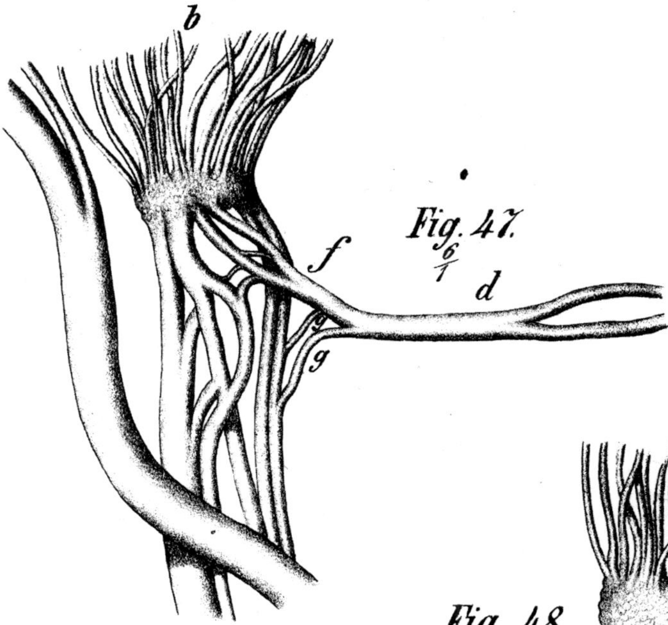

Fig. 47. $\frac{6}{1}$

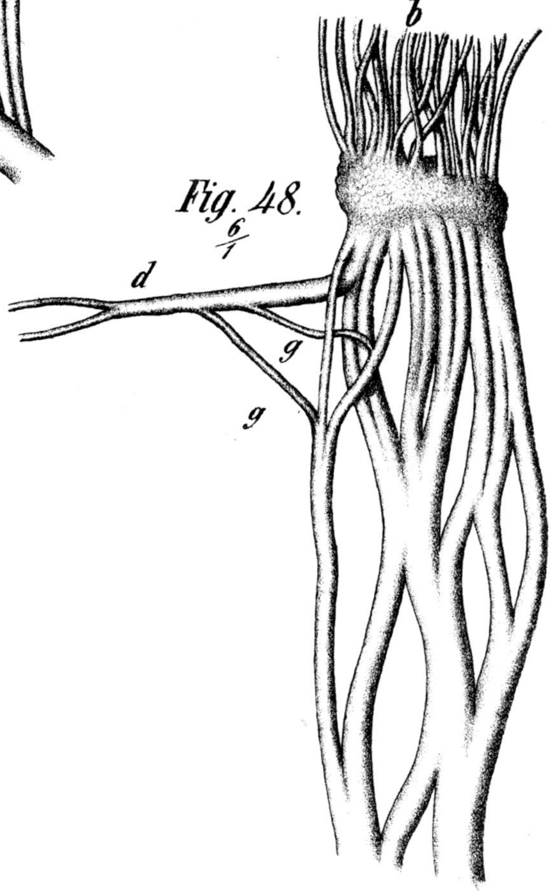

Fig. 48. $\frac{6}{1}$

Fig. 46. c. $\frac{6}{1}$

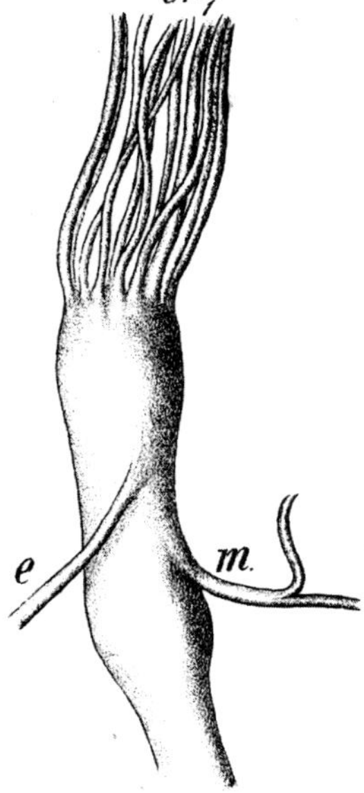

Fig. 49.
6/1

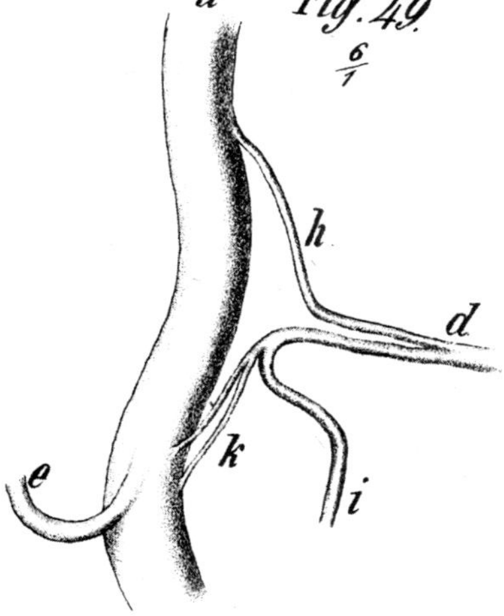

Fig. 50.
6/1

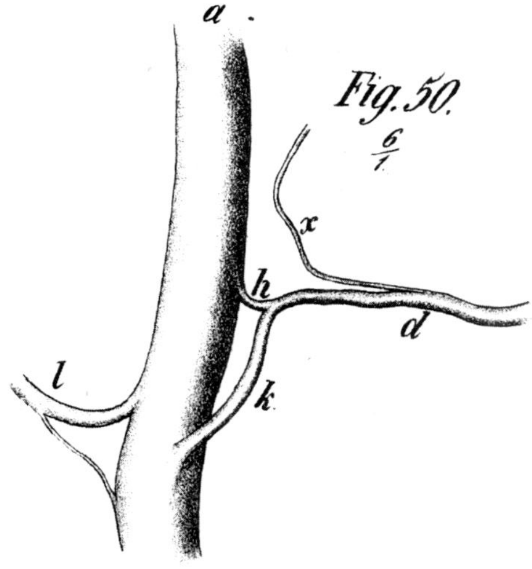

the auricular nerve. However, Longet too (pp. 206, 360) mentions this connection from the facial to the auricular nerve, and therefore calls the latter a mixed nerve, but without stating in what direction the branches go. Sappey, on the other hand, has a very different conception (pp. 259, 287, 279, and figure 220, p. 300). According to him the trunk of the auricular branch of the vagus consists of two nerves; one which starts from the [superior—*ed.*] jugular ganglion and follows the path as described by Arnold; it also forms an anastomosis with the facial nerve, and disappears at the ear drum; another starts at the facial nerve and takes a retrograde course toward the jugular ganglion of the vagus nerve. In addition, Sappey shows in his figure a branch going from the trunk of the auricular nerve to the [inferior—*ed.*] petrosal ganglion of the glossopharyngeal nerve. Finally, he describes an anastomosis between the facial and the glossopharyngeal nerve, and states that this anastomosis is frequently missing; but if it occurs, it goes immediately after leaving the stylomastoid foramen to the glossopharyngeal nerve underneath the petrosal ganglion. I mention this here because Sappey does not speak about the origin of the auricular nerve from the glossopharyngeal nerve.

I must admit that I had great difficulties with the preparation and study of this part of the nervous system and that in spite of repeated experiments I did not reach a complete understanding of some of the points, not only because of the difficulties involved, but also because the course of the auricular nerve varies in different individuals.

As far as the origin of the auricular branch of the vagus nerve is concerned, we must know the direction of its small composite strands to understand its course; it originates, as stated by Arnold, from the vagus as well as from the glossopharyngeal nerve. In regard to the vagus, it always comes out of one or several nerve bundles coming from the jugular ganglion and is centrally located, which means that the fibers are derived from the vagus. The study of the glossopharyngeal origin is more complicated. It starts above the petrosal ganglion and beneath the jugular ganglion of this nerve, which is between the two. The rootlets of the glossopharyngeal also come mostly from the center and go therefore from the glossopharyngeal to the auricular branch of the vagus nerve. However, I saw several times on the vagus, as well as the glossopharyngeal, how fibers of this root of the auricular branch of the vagus turn off at the periphery—an indication that they passed from one nerve to the other. In cases where I did not notice this, it is quite probable that because of the difficulty of the experiment I overlooked those small rootlets, or that they were torn off during the preparation. In addition, the origin from the glossopharyngeal nerve shows a number of discrepancies. I believe that sometimes the nerve does not exist at all, or perhaps is extremely thin. Sometimes the thread of the glossopharyngeal nerve involved does not directly join the root of the vagus, but merges with the trunk of this latter nerve, from which that root of the auricular nerve leaves. This means that in fact an anastomosis exists here between glossopharyngeal and vagus, although probably in the root of the vagus its fibers separate again toward the auricular nerve [Figures 53-63].

The study of the course of the nerve in the jugular fossa is relatively easy, particularly if this fossa is sufficiently wide, as is usually the case on the right side. Several times, although not always, I could recognize beyond any doubt that at this point the nerve consisted of two rootlets that, throughout their course, were separated only at certain points.

It is extremely difficult to demonstrate and to study the entry of the nerve into the Fallopian canal, the continuation of its connection with the facial nerve, and especially its further course through the so-called mastoid canaliculus. The connection with the facial nerve does by no means occur through strands as distinct, strong, and long as one is inclined to believe when looking at figures by Arnold, Beck, and others. On the contrary, the trunk of the auricular nerve runs very close alongside the facial nerve and even passes through the latter's sheath. The connecting twigs with the facial nerve lie within this sheath and are so thin that they can be recognized only after the sheath has been made clearer by means of acetic acid and under an illuminated magnifying glass, and mostly with the help of compression.

I always saw that a small branch descends from the posterior edge of the facial nerve and approaches the auricular nerve from the back, thus going from the former to the latter. All scientists working on this problem have apparently seen this strand, which Longet and Sappey have called "anastomosis of the facial nerve with the pneumogastric nerve." However, nobody says where he supposes this branch of the facial nerve is going peripherally. It may possibly pass into the jugular ganglion of the vagus or the glossopharyngeal nerve and form a connection between that ganglion with the facial nerve. But if I am right in what I believe I have seen, namely that the beginning of the auricular nerve from the glossopharyngeal and the vagus also has fibers that run peripherally, it follows that the strand of the facial nerve in these nerves could also run peripherally. Probably, as has sometimes been recognized, this observation can also be applied to the fact that during its course across the jugular fossa the auricular nerve is composed of two strands, and therefore Sappey is right when he maintains that it consists of two nerves running in opposite directions.

FIGURES 53 TO 63

These figures are meant to show the relations of the tympanic, the lesser superficial petrosal and Jacobson's anastomosis in the tympanic cavity. Everywhere I have drawn the relations of the first two nerves, as if fibers run from the lesser superficial petrosal or from the otic ganglion to the glossopharyngeal nerve, as well as fibers from the tympanic nerve to the otic ganglion. Because of the peripheral course of several fibers of the tympanic trunk in the glossopharyngeal nerve, the first situation is absolutely certain; the second, however, can only be surmised from the thickness of the tympanic nerve and the nerves derived from it. It must be concluded that a number of fibers remain, which can only lie in the course of the lesser superficial petrosal.

a glossopharyngeal nerve

b facial nerve

c tympanic nerve

d lesser superficial petrosal

e nerves going to the round window

f caroticotympanic nerve, the lesser deep petrosal

g nerves belonging to the Eustachian tube

h ganglion at the lesser superficial petrosal which I discovered

i nerve to the oval window

k small artery between the lesser superficial petrosal and the genu of the facial nerve which erroneously was believed to be an anastomosis between the two nerves.

l greater superficial petrosal nerve

[o strand ascending from lesser superficial petrosal to carotid plexus. *Ed.*]

Figure 53. A very complete preparation showing the following: (1) The peripheral course of several fibers of the tympanic nerve at its origin from the glossopharyngeal nerve. (2) The ganglion observed by me at the nerve to the oval window and in addition a second ganglion at the trunk of the lesser superficial petrosal. (3) The fibers of the caroticotympanic nerve very definitely going from the carotid into the tympanic cavity and then, without further spreading out, into the Eustachian tube. (4) As all other preparations without exception have shown, no anastomosis exists between the genu of the facial nerve and the lesser superficial petrosal, but a small artery has the appearance of such a connection.

Figure 54. Here the peripheral entrance of several fibers of the tympanic into the trunk of the glossopharyngeal nerve was very clear. But in regard to (f) and (g) the preparation was probably turned around when it was taken out, so that the caroticotympanic nerve was situated on top. It also seems dubious whether the nerve at (e) goes only to the round window, because it is too strong and composed of strands that enter from above and below.

Figure 55. This preparation is notable because the course of the fibers does not cause sympathetic nerves to enter the anastomosis, but the strands (f) go to the carotid, or more likely spread out in the chorda tympani too. The small ganglion (h) seems unusual, inasmuch as it is connected with the lesser superficial petrosal merely through a very small strand, although usually it lies very close to the petrosal.

Figure 56 is very unusual in regard to the course of the fibers of the caroticotympanic nerve (f), since after having approached the trunk of the tympanic, the nerve merges immediately with the nerve for the Eustachian tube.

Figure 57. A trunk of the glossopharyngeal nerve stripped of its sheath; the trunk of the tympanic nerve consists of two strands almost from the start. Numerous nerves leave the ganglion of the petrosal, of which some have probably brought about the connection with the vagus nerve, and another one may be the root for the auricular nerve. The others are unknown to me.

Figure 58 shows a remarkable split of the trunk of the tympanic nerve, and a course just as remarkable and unusual as the caroticotympanic nerve. Possibly one strand passes from the glossopharyngeal nerve into the plexus of the carotid, although my picture shows it the other way around. It is equally dubious whether the strand (o) ascends from the lesser superficial petrosal into the plexus of the carotid.

Figure 59. This preparation is unusual because of the arrangement of its strands:

1. The large nerve at (e) for the round window.
2. The exit occurring at such a height of the nerves to the tympanic tube (g) and their course into the carotid canal (f).
3. The sole exit of fibers of the tympanic nerve into the Eustachian tube.

Finally, the passage of the sympathetic fiber (f) into the lesser superficial petrosal seems unusual unless we want to assume that it passes from the latter into the plexus of the carotid. In the last two cases I did not find a ganglion for the oval window at the nerve (i).

Figure 60 shows again a trunk of the tympanic nerve split from the beginning and the passage of one of its branches to the plexus of the carotid—or vice versa. In addition, there occurs the passage of sympathetic nerves to the lesser superficial petrosal or vice versa, and an involvement of sympathetic fibers in the nerves of the Eustachian tube.

Figure 61 is notable only because of its position and the high exit of the nerves to the Eustachian tube and from the plexus of the carotid. At this point the latter goes only to the Eustachian tube.

Figures 62 and 63. Two drawings of the tympanic plexus, which are special inasmuch as the nerves were drawn first when they were still in their position in the tympanic cavity so that no mixups could happen. Only afterward were they taken out and the course of the fibers studied.

Figure 62 is remarkable because of the thickness of the lesser deep petrosal (f), which I have pictured with all its fibers originating from the plexus of the carotid and running toward the petrosal as well as the ganglion, but also to the area of the round window. The nerve (i) went to the area of the oval window (a), although not in a straight line; perhaps the true nerve for this point was only a branch. A ganglion could not be detected.

Figure 63 is particularly important because it shows that the lesser superficial petrosal (d) is not involved in the formation of any nerves of the Eustachian tube, but goes only from the otic ganglion to the petrous ganglion. In contrast, the tympanic nerve is very strongly developed. Almost all those nerves go to the Eustachian tube (g), and there is only one very fine strand (i) from which two very small ganglia go to the oval window. Here the lesser deep petrosal goes only to the sheath and the ganglion of the petrosal nerve.

Fig. 53.

$\frac{6}{1}$

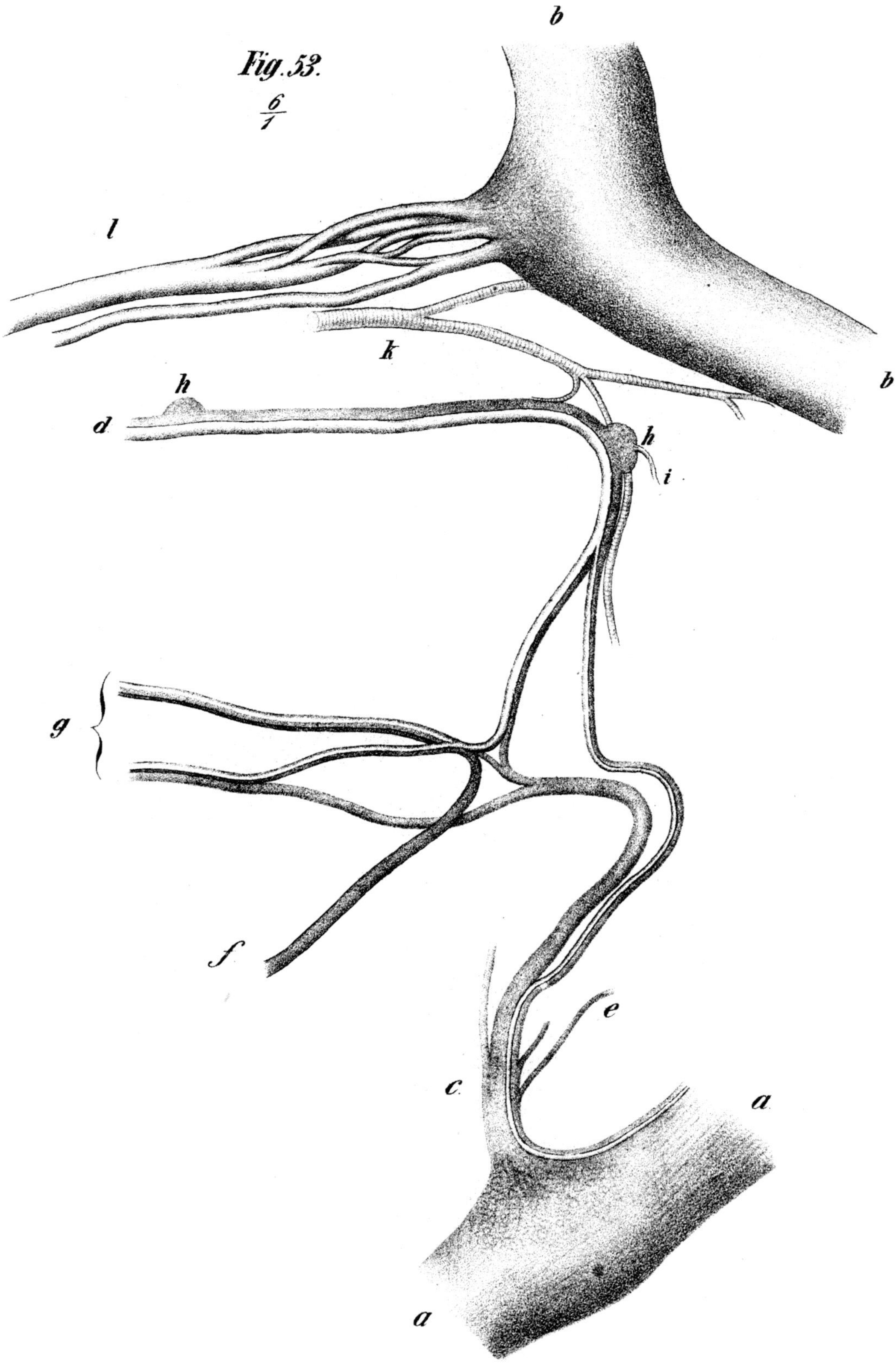

Fig. 54.

$\frac{6}{1}$ b.

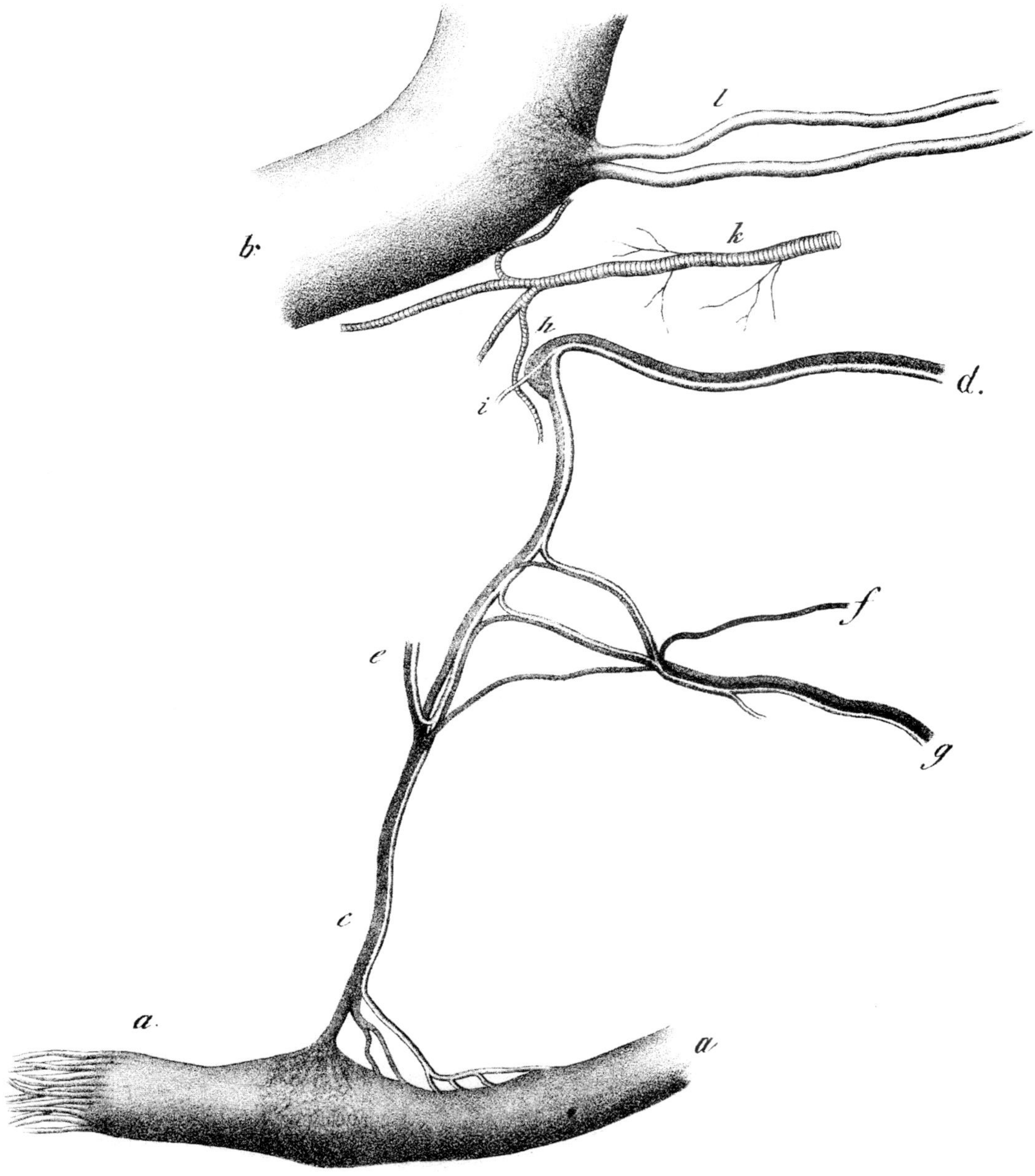

Fig. 55.

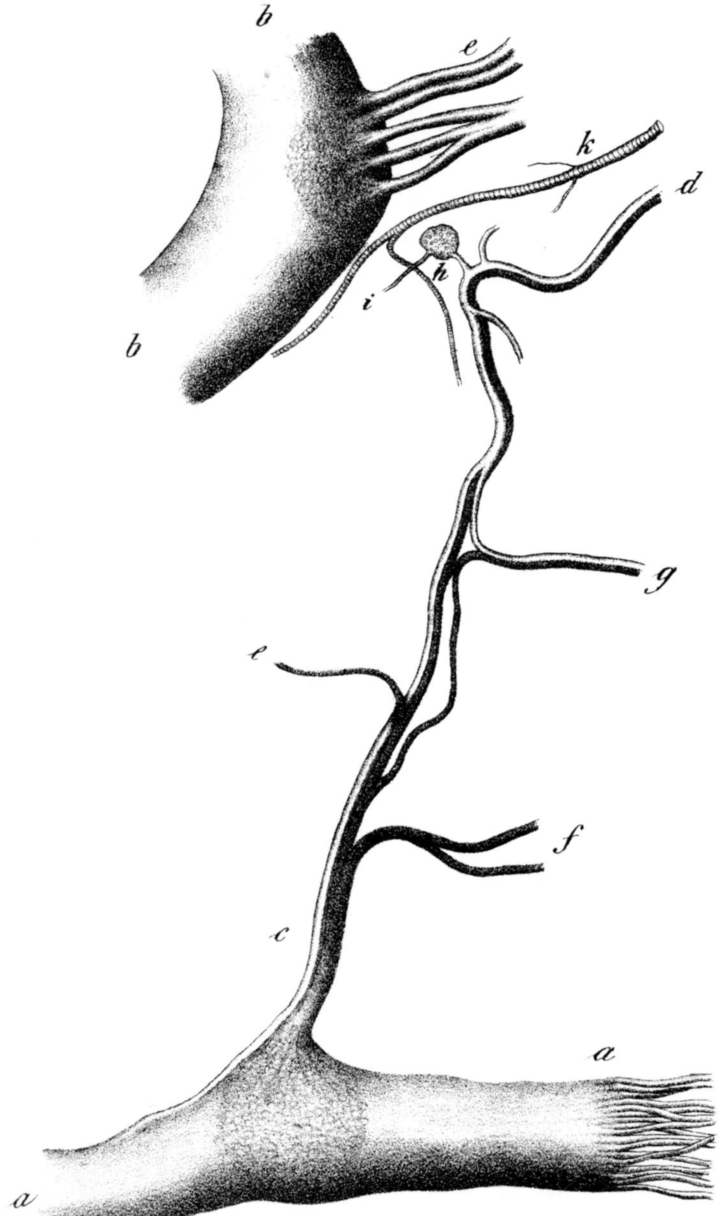

Fig. 56.

$\frac{4}{1}$

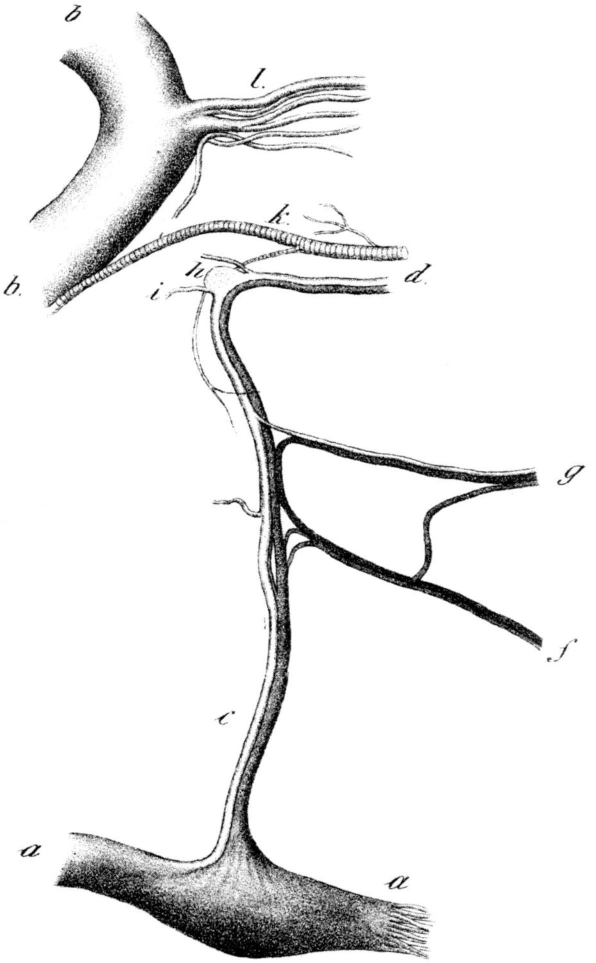

Fig. 57.

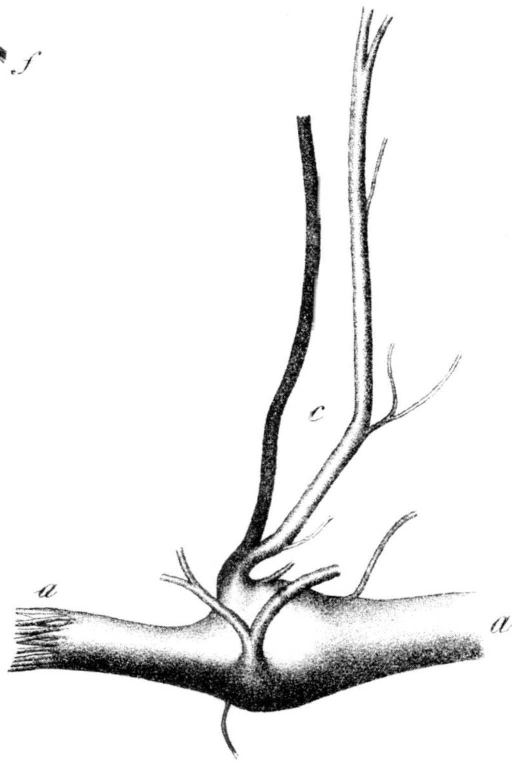

Fig. 58.

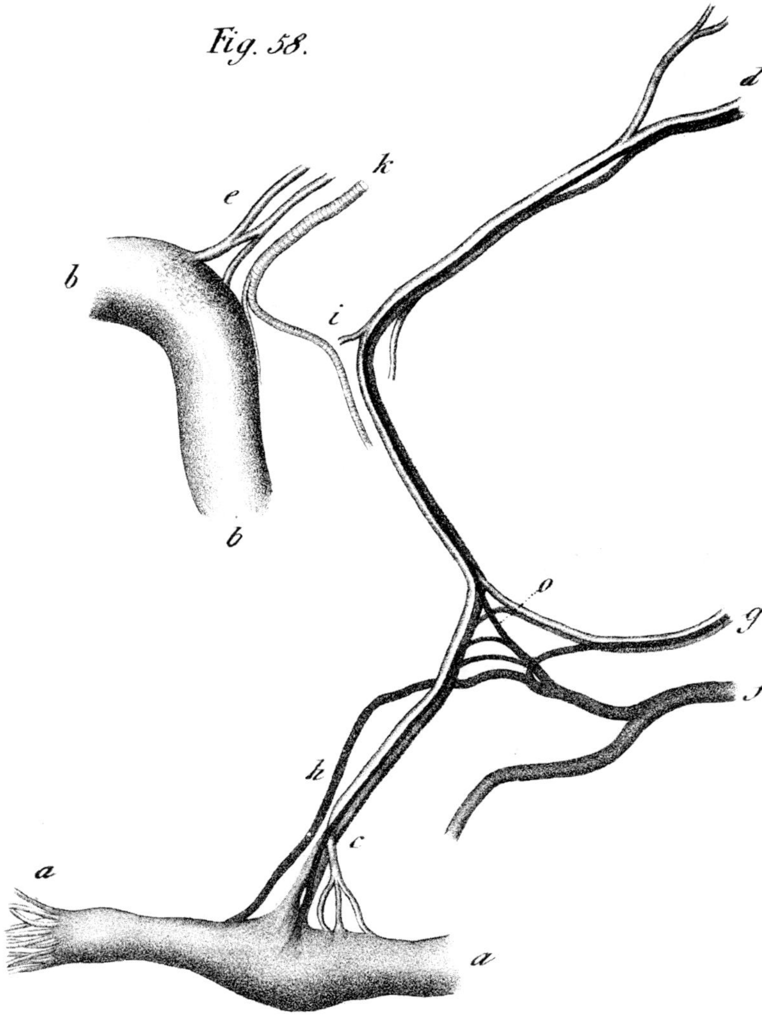

Fig. 59.

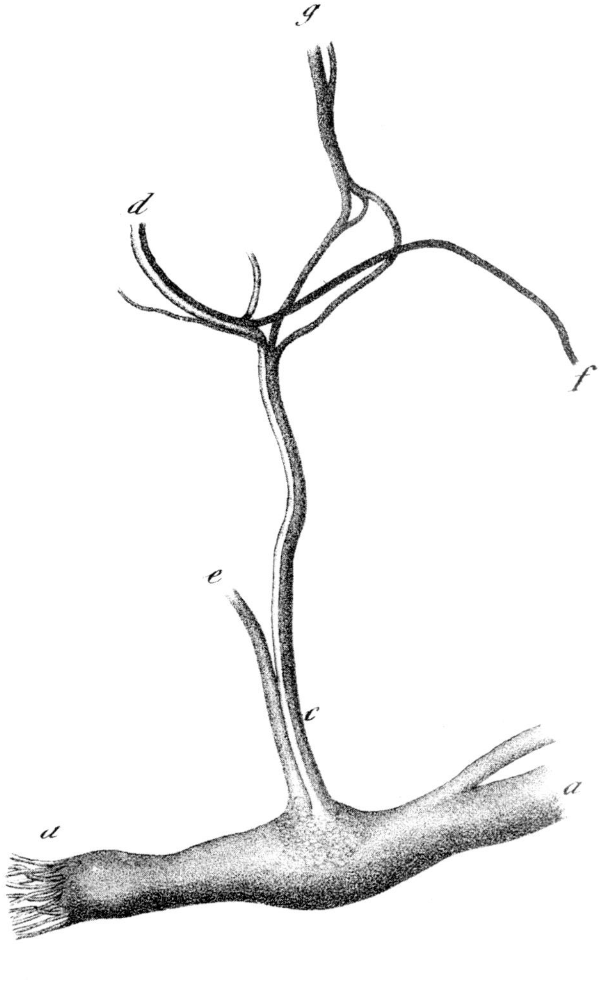

Fig. 60.
6/1

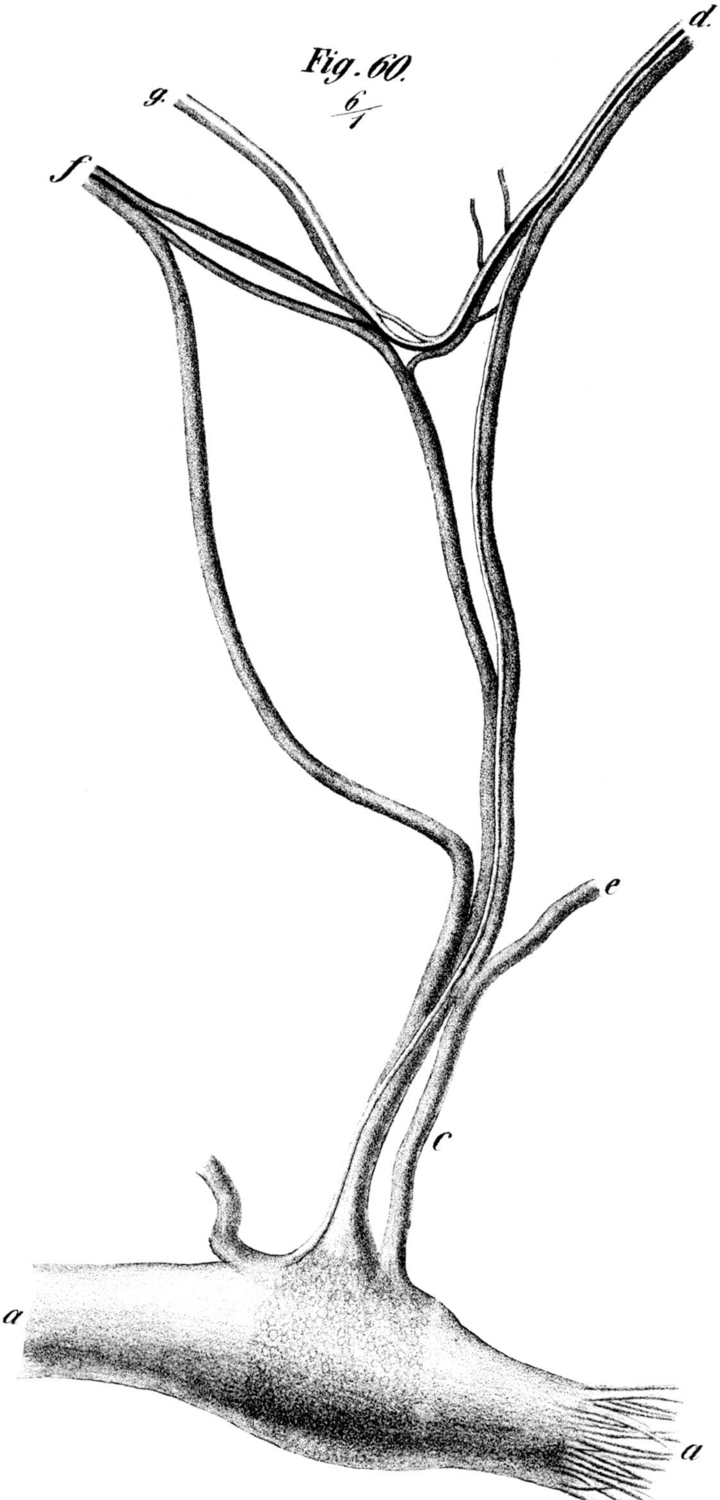

Fig. 61.
6/1

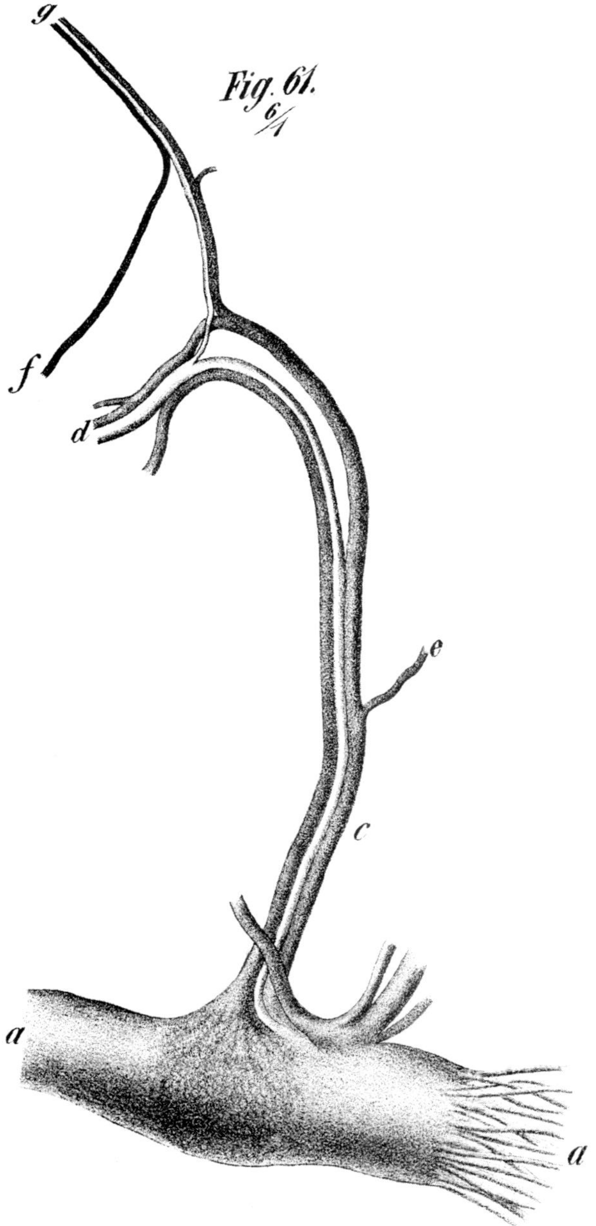

Fig. 62.
6/1

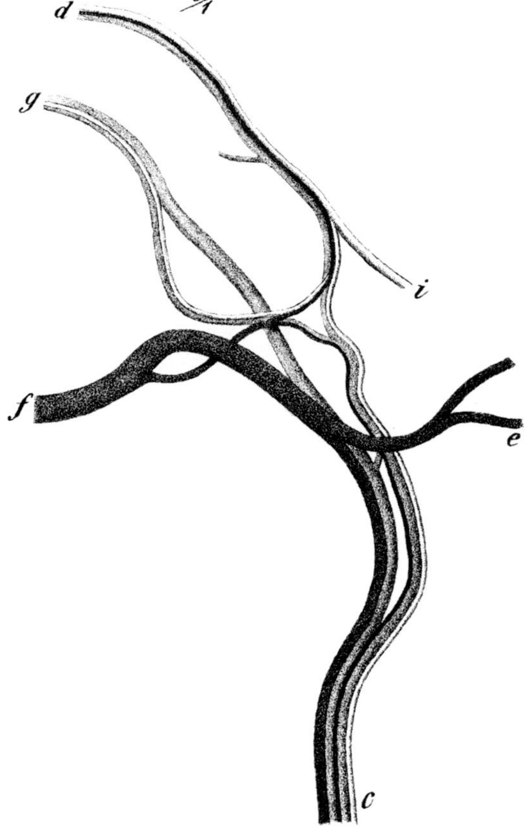

Fig. 63.

6/1

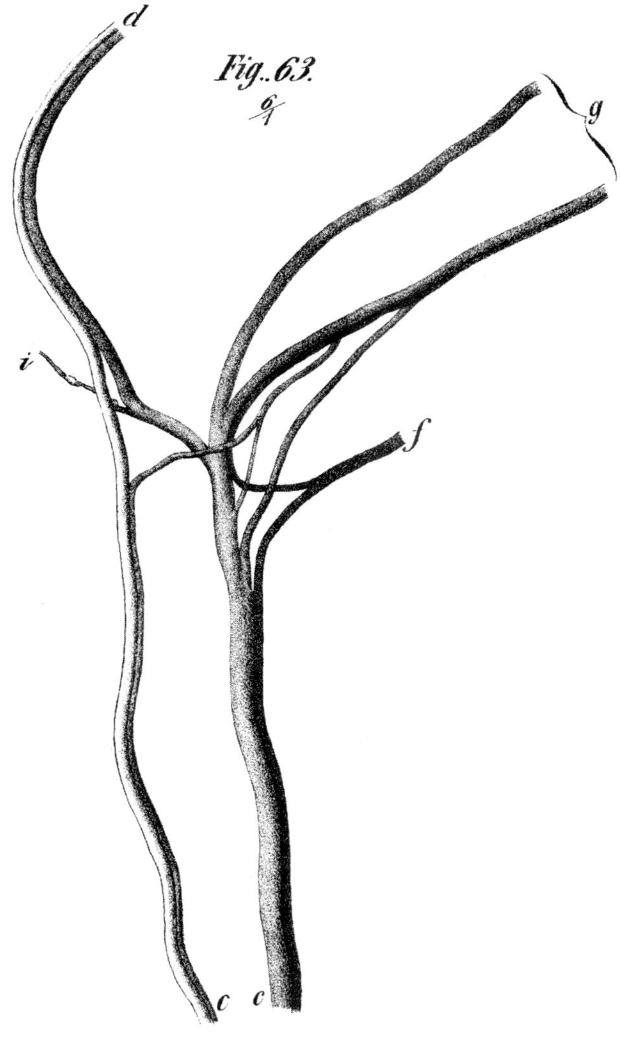

We will now discuss the question of the second connection of the auricular branch with the facial nerve, namely the one that descends from the auricular to the facial nerve. This connection, too, certainly exists sometimes, since I am sure that I have seen more than once how the auricular, when it had reached the facial nerve, was divided into three branches: the one we have just discussed, ascending toward the facial nerve; one that descends; and one in the middle which runs across the facial nerve and forms the continuation of the trunk into the mastoid canaliculus. It seems to me, however, that the connection descending to the facial nerve rarely occurs; usually I did not see it. It is therefore understandable that some authors, like Arnold, believe it is a regular feature. Occasionally the auricular nerve, instead of splitting into two terminal branches after its passage through the Fallopian canal, does so before it enters the canal. After that the upper branch goes straight across the facial nerve, takes in the strand that descends from the facial nerve, and runs in the opposite direction; then it goes through the mastoid canaliculus behind the ear. The lower branch, on the other hand, slants downward and across the facial nerve into the latter's sheath; this is the second terminal branch of the auricular nerve, which joins the deep auricular branch of the facial nerve outside the stylomastoid foramen. It can easily happen that the latter will be erroneously regarded as the anastomosis which descends from the auricular to the facial nerve; this error has been made more than once, since it is not easy to follow this very fine nerve beyond the Fallopian canal.

Besides the foregoing I also venture to state that sometimes the auricular branch of the vagus nerve merges completely with the facial nerve, and that its trunk runs peripherally. Then it probably leaves the latter again in the deep auricular branch of the facial nerve. For not only did I try several times in vain to find the continuation of the auricular nerve through a mastoid calaliculus, but after eliminating the sheath of the nerve I distinctly detected this passage of the auricular into the path of the facial nerve.

I also think that I can vouch for the possibility of a reverse situation—namely, that the auricular branch of the vagus may not join the facial at all, neither through a descending nor an ascending branch. [True, but he wasn't sure. *Ed.*] Several times I have seen it rather strongly developed, separated into two strands, encased in the sheath of the facial nerve and passing across the latter without my being able to detect a connecting strand, even though my study was extremely meticulous and I had made the parts more transparent with acetic acid, had split them, and had carefully pulled them off under the magnifying glass.

Perhaps my findings will meet with doubts when I say that sometimes the auricular branch of the vagus does not exist at all. But through very frequent preparations I have gained so much practice in following its path, and it can so easily be found in the jugular fossa, that I cannot imagine that I ever overlooked it unless it could be reduced to an extremely thin strand. [More probably the latter. *Ed.*]

As for the connections that the facial nerve partially forms with the branches of the second and third divisions of the trigeminal nerve after having left the stylomastoid foramen, and partially with the nerves of the neck, I have thoroughly examined only the anastomoses between the auriculo-temporal nerve of the third division of the trigeminal nerve and the branches of the facial nerve which are located underneath and in front of the external auditory canal [Figures 51, 52]. This anastomosis is formed with the help of several strong branches of both nerves. Few anatomists (e.g., Arnold, p. 871) furnish exact descriptions of the manner in which the connection of the two nerves takes place, although most of them seem to assume that sensory fibers of the auriculo-temporal nerve are transported to the facial nerve through this anastomosis. This is indeed exclusively the case. Two to four branches of the auriculo-temporal nerve go close to the plexi of the facial nerve, and most of them pass—although not entirely and not in every case—into their sheaths and together with them spread out peripherally. The opposite—that is, passage of fibers of the facial nerve into the path of the auriculo-temporal nerve—never occurs.

The same is true of the points of connection between the facial nerve and the infraorbital nerve of the second division, as well as the mental nerve of the third division of the trigeminal nerve and, finally, of branches of the upper nerves of the neck. Everywhere the fibers of both nerves approach one another closely through single branches and disperse in the skin and the muscles.

Finally, it appears that the anastomosis mentioned by most anatomists, although not as a constant one between the digastric ramus of the facial nerve and the branch with the same name of the glossopharyngeal nerve [Figures 64-66], apparently has an arc shape of fibers going from the one nerve to the other. As a matter of fact, however, each of the two rami seemingly going away from each other is usually divided into two branches, which alternately approach each other closely but then continue peripherally. Sometimes the situation is not that simple, and it seems that we are faced with an "anastomosis without end." There can be no doubt, however, that there are branches higher up which leave the trunks peripherally in a central direction. [For instance, Figure 65 shows the branch leaving the facial nerve at least on one side. *Ed.*]

FIGURES 51 AND 52

Figures 51 and 52 show the anastomosis between the facial and the auriculotemporal branch of V^3. The branches of the two nerves run alongside each other in order to make the connection, and they spread out at the periphery.

a facial nerve

b auriculotemporal branch of V^3

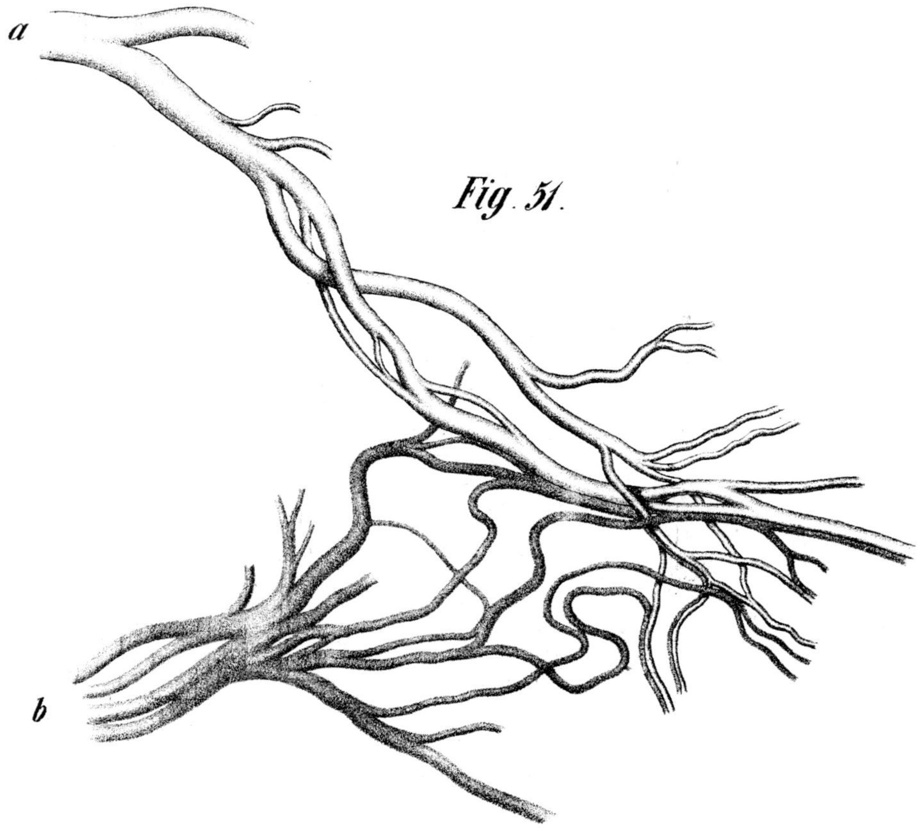

Fig. 52.

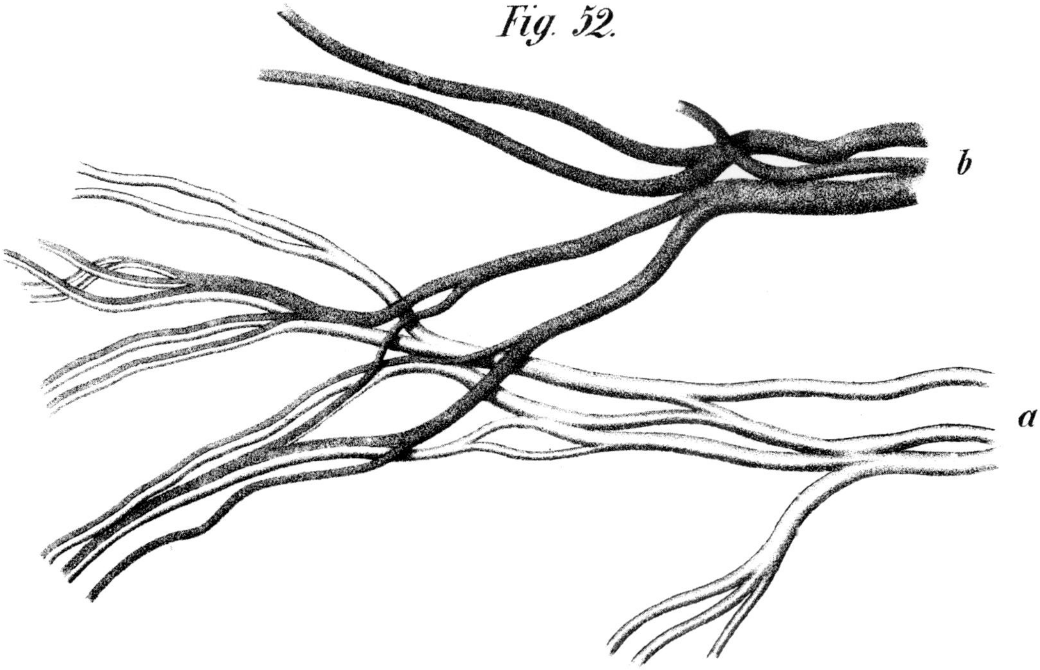

FIGURES 64 TO 66

Figure 64 shows an anastomosis between the digastric ramus of the facial nerve and that of the glossopharyngeal nerve. In this preparation I found, despite a thorough study, no trace of the auricular branch of the vagus, either at the vagus or at the facial nerve, or in the jugular fossa.

a vagus nerve

b glossopharyngeal nerve

c facial nerve

d digastric ramus of the glossopharyngeal nerve

e digastric ramus of the facial nerve

f perhaps a small root of an insignificant auricular branch of the vagus nerve

g tympanic nerve

h deep auricular ramus of the facial nerve

Figure 65 shows the same anastomosis between the digastric ramus of the facial nerve and the glossopharyngeal nerve—as being apparently without end. Only at the digastric ramus of the facial nerve we see at (i) a thread running in a central direction, which without doubt originates from the glossopharyngeal nerve. Probably a similar strand originating from the facial nerve existed at the digastric ramus of the glossopharyngeal nerve; however, this strand separated further up and therefore was not noticed.

Figure 66 shows an apparent anastomosis without end between the pharyngeal ramus of the vagus (a) and the pharyngeal ramus of the glossopharyngeal nerve (b).

Fig. 64.

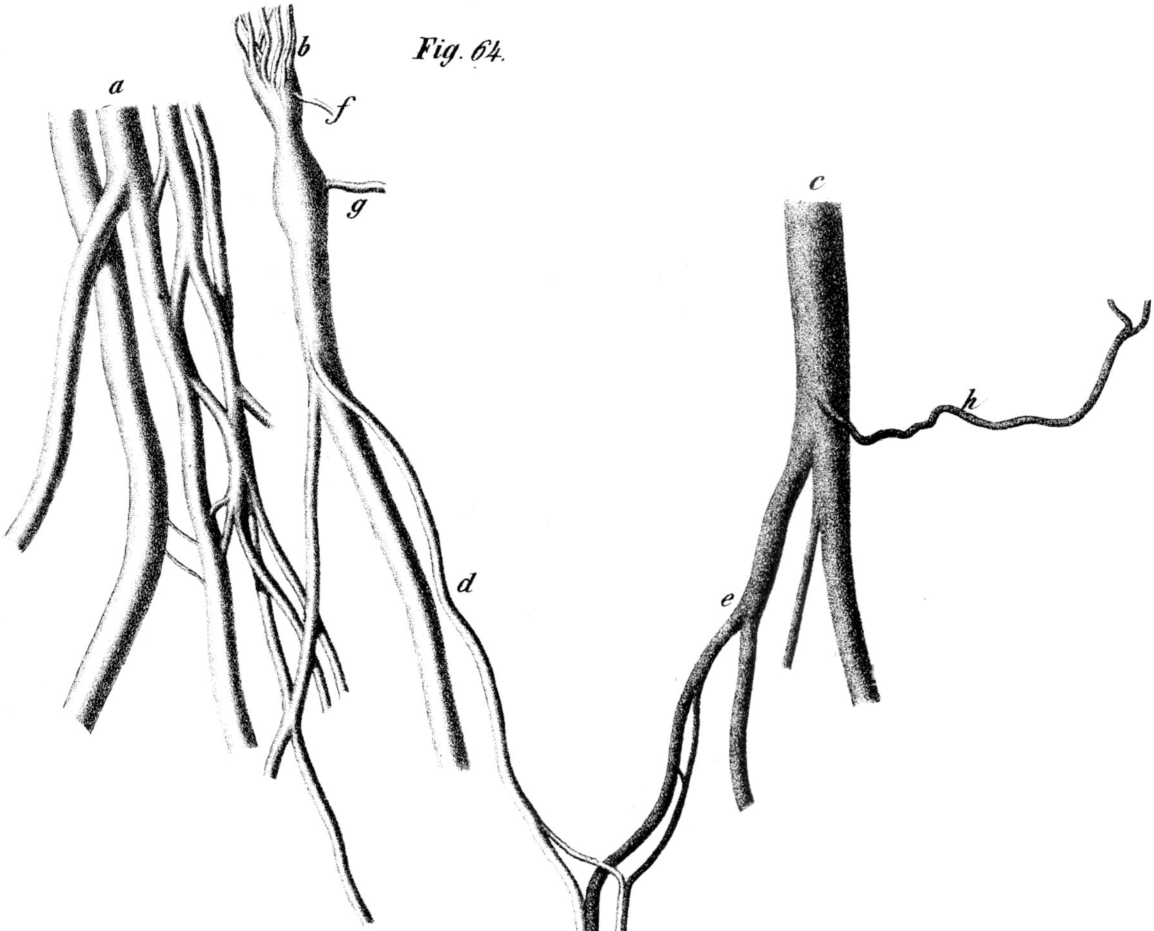

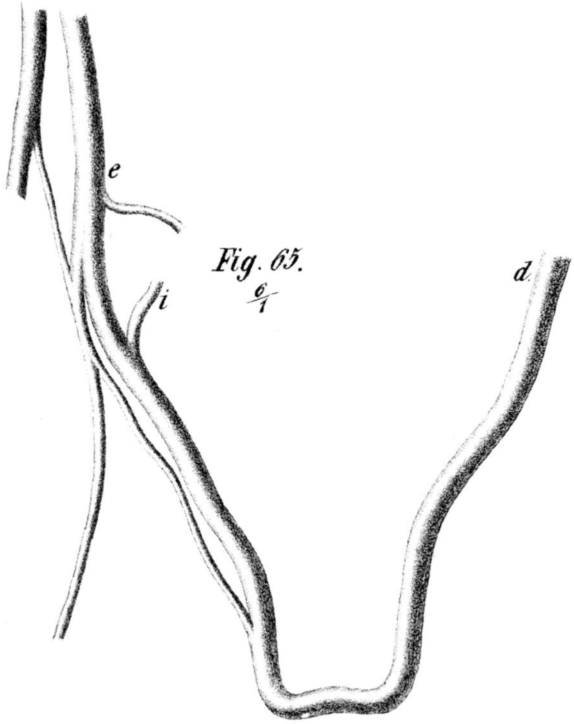

Fig. 65.
6/1

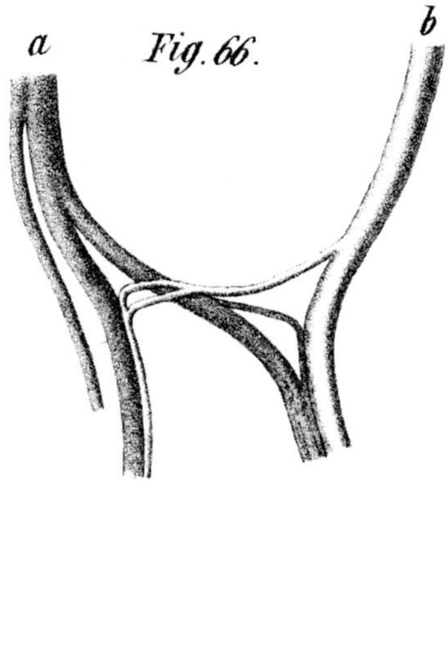

Fig. 66.

V. The Glossopharyngeal Nerve

As far as the glossopharyngeal nerve is concerned, I have mainly studied its tympanic ramus and its anastomosis—known as Jacobson's anastomosis—with several nerves on the inner wall of the tympanic cavity. But it should be noted that immediately after having left the jugular foramen, the glossopharyngeal nerve also enters into a connection with its neighbor the vagus nerve. The twig that brings about this connection usually comes out of the petrosal ganglion, but it is very short and seems to go from the glossopharyngeal to the vagus nerve. Sometimes small connecting branches can also be found further down; but since this occurs only rarely, those branches are of no particular importance. Frequently an anastomosis also appears between the pharyngeal ramus of the glossopharyngeal nerve and the branch of the same name from the vagus, which, judging by its outward appearance, could be assumed to be one of those anastomoses without end [Figures 67–70]. But more meticulous observations show that the branches of both nerves approach each other so closely that they form a plexus, from which the peripheral ramifications originate.

A well known anastomosis is Jacobson's anastomosis of the tympanic ramus of the glossopharyngeal nerve, which we have mentioned above and which has been explored frequently.

I believe that I should not go into a detailed description of the background of its discovery and study, since that has already been done numerous times earlier, particularly by Beck in his paper on the seventh and ninth pair of the cranial nerves. I will therefore confine myself to the discussion of those findings which are still taught at the present time and are connected with the results of my study. In that respect only two doctrines have to be considered.

One of those opinions is Arnold's, with whom Beck agrees. According to them, the above-mentioned plexus [of the IX and X—*ed.*] is merely composed of the ramifications of the tympanic nerve which leave the petrosal ganglion and enter the tympanic cavity. Besides sending one or more twigs into the Eustachian tube as well as to the oval window and the cells of the retromastoid process, the tympanic nerve sends one or two branches, the deep

FIGURES 67 TO 70

Here we see the trunks of the glossopharyngeal, the vagus, the spinal accessory nerve of Willis, and the hypoglossal nerve. This figure serves as a demonstration of an anastomosis between the pharyngeal ramus of the glossopharyngeal nerve and the pharyngeal ramus of the vagus; the major part of the former comes from the internal ramus of the spinal accessory nerve of Willis.

a glossopharyngeal nerve

b vagus nerve

c spinal accessory nerve of Willis

d hypoglossal nerve

e anastomosis between the two pharyngeal rami of the vagus and the glossopharyngeal nerve

g branch of the first cervical nerve going to the hypoglossal nerve

Figure 67. Although for the most part the anastomosis is only an apparent one, there seem to be loops without end at e, f, and i. The auricular of the vagus originates with two roots from the glossopharyngeal nerve and with three roots from the vagus, and it is very strong.

Figure 68. Here the entire anastomosis is only an apparent one, and through the branch (k) it brings about a connection between the trunks of the glossopharyngeal and the vagus. The auricular nerve of the vagus originates with only one root from the vagus, and it is weak.

Figure 69. This figure shows the connection of the glossopharyngeal nerve with the vagus: (a) the glossopharyngeal nerve; "bbb" three bundles of the vagus, from one of which the auricular of the vagus originates with two split roots; (d) the connection between glossopharyngeal and vagus that comes about through several strands, most of which go from the latter to the former. But (d) also includes strands of the glossopharyngeal nerve, probably running toward a second strand of the vagus (e).

Figure 70. Another case of a connection between the glossopharyngeal nerve (b) and the vagus (a) a bit further down through the strands (cc).

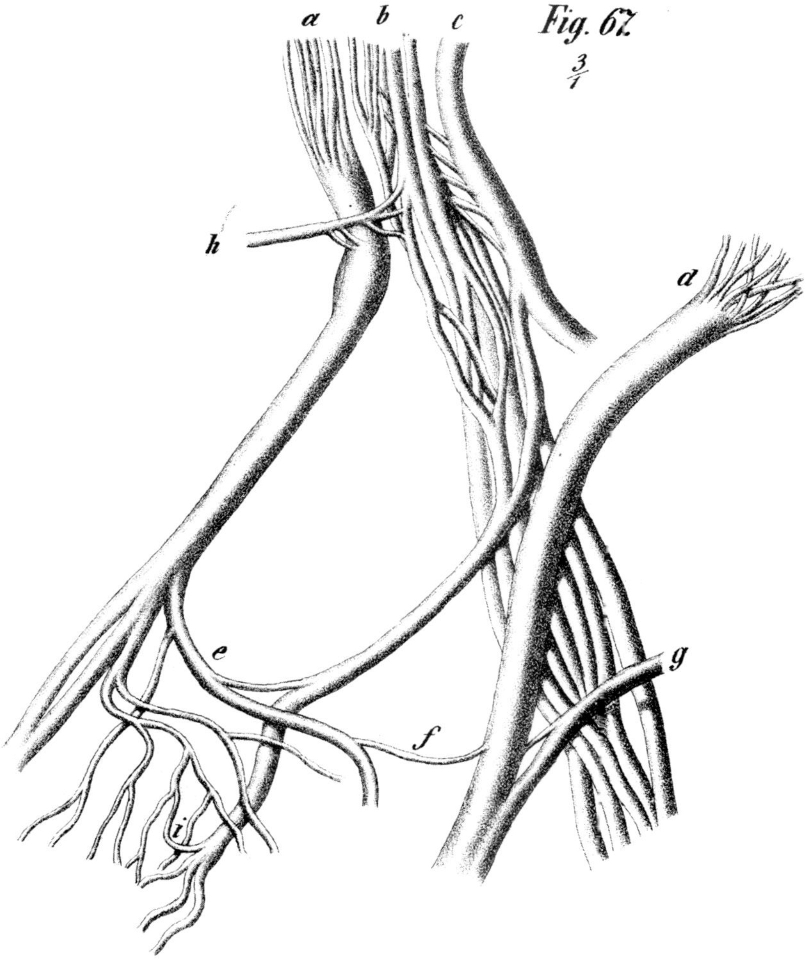

Fig. 67.
3/1

Fig. 68.

$\frac{3}{1}$

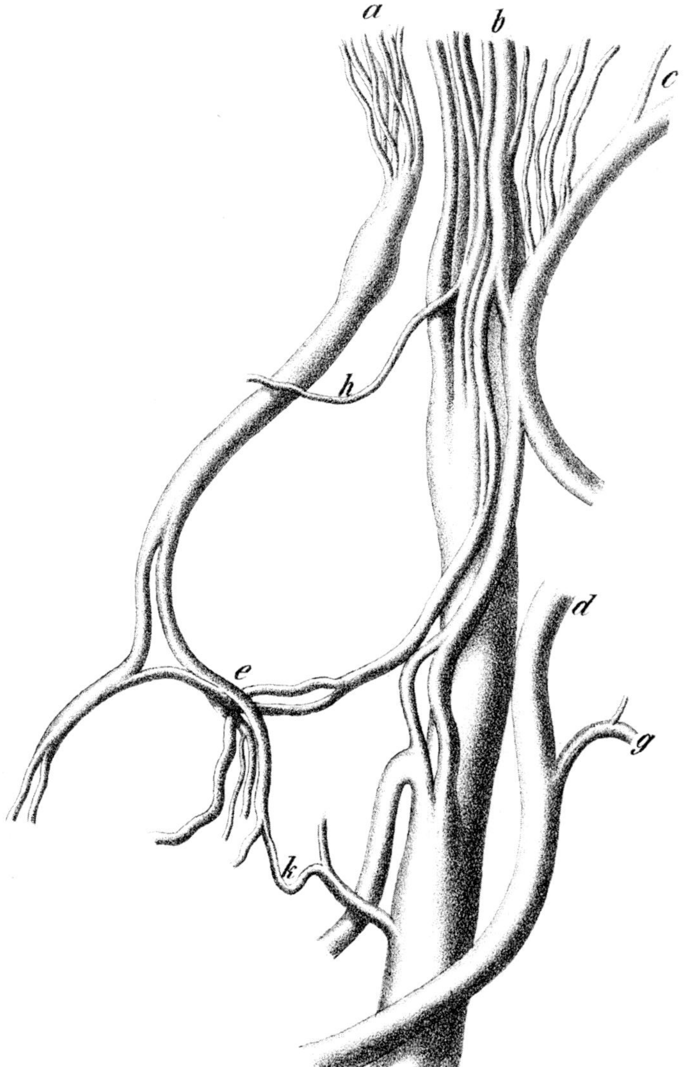

Fig. 69.
6/1

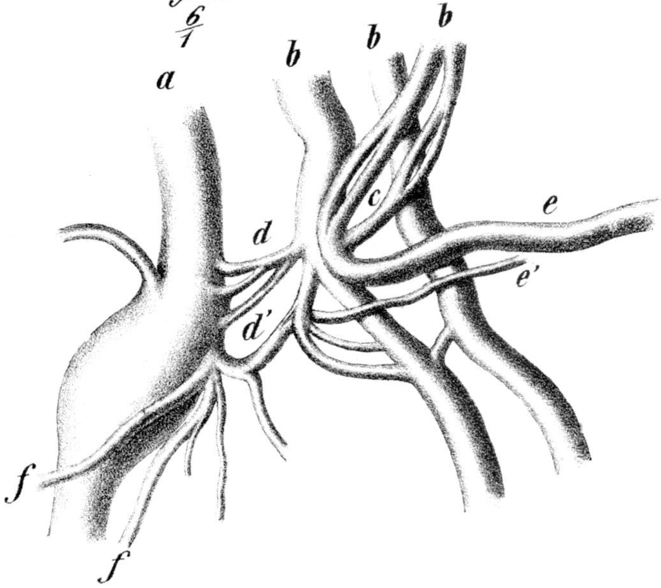

Fig. 70.
3/1

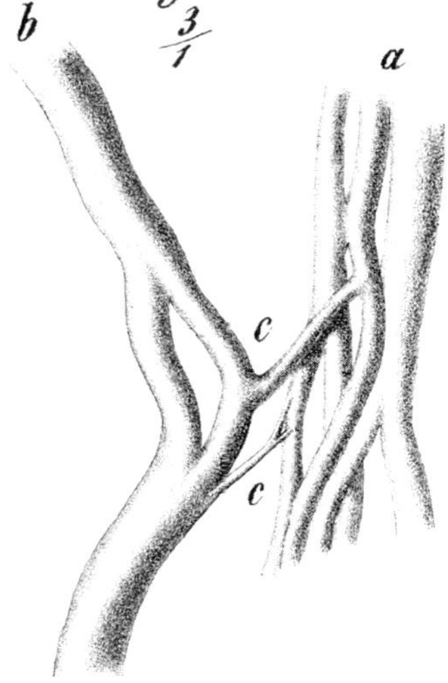

minor nerves, through small openings in the anterior wall of the tympanic cavity into the carotid canal, where they merge with the carotid nerve. The real continuation of the nerve, its terminal branch, ascends within a groove on the promontory to the cranial cavity, reaches the upper petrosal level through its special canaliculus between the Fallopian canal and the tympanic sulcus tensoris, then turns outward to the front of the greater superficial petrosal and through a small hole between the foramen spinosum and foramen ovale, where it reaches the otic ganglion at the posterior level of the third branch of the trigeminal nerve. Arnold, who discovered this branch, called it the lesser superficial petrosal and regarded it as the long or sensory root of the above-mentioned ganglion, which consequently is being supplied by the glossopharyngeal nerve.

Krause, Valentin, Hyrtl, and others are of a very different opinion. According to them a genuine anastomosis develops at the promontory of the tympanic cavity, formed by the tympanic nerve originating from the glossopharyngeal nerve as well as the sympathetic branches coming from the carotid canal, the so-called lesser deep petrosal nerve, and finally a nerve, the lesser superficial petrosal, coming from the otic ganglion and penetrating into the tympanic cavity. These scientists believe that—in a manner not further explained—a number of strands separate from this anastomosis and run toward the oval window, the cells of the mastoid process and the Eustachian tube.

In addition almost all authors indicate unanimously that a small connective twig goes to the genu of the facial nerve from the lesser superficial petrosal at the point where it runs between the Fallopian canal and the tympanic sulcus tensoris; some believe that it goes from the lesser superficial petrosal to the facial nerve, while others believe it to be vice versa. Longet, who agrees with the latter opinion, assumes this small branch which originates from the facial nerve to be the motor root of the otic ganglion. Beck is the only one who has up to now disavowed the existence of the branch and claims that it is a small artery.

As is well known, the preparation of this segment of nerve is one of the most difficult. The nerves are thin and for the most part run through small bony canals or within bony grooves; consequently, it is hard to separate them. On the other hand, it is easy to see certain parts, particularly on the inner side of the tympanic nerve, after they have been swabbed with acetic acid. In spite of these difficulties and after a great number of experiments, I succeeded in separating the segments intact, after the nerves had been rendered clearer by treating them with acetic acid, compressed with the help of the compressor and greatly enlarged under the microscope. I believe that thus I was able to analyze their course more exactly than my predecessors.

As far as the origin of the tympanic nerve from the petrosal [inferior-ganglion—*ed.*] of the glossopharyngeal nerve is concerned, although there can be no doubt that most of its fibers originate from the ganglion and are probably connected with the ganglion, they cannot be followed up to the fibers of the glossopharyngeal nerve. But I am sure that in several cases I saw how some of the fibers did not form a connection with the ganglion, but descended into the peripheral segment of the glossopharyngeal nerve and, according to the direction of their entrance, continued to the periphery of this nerve. In addition, it sometimes happens that the trunk of the tympanic nerve is double. Although its two strands lie very close together, they are distinctly two separate branches and probably have a different origin. This will be seen in our further discussion.

Regarding the origin of the lesser superficial petrosal nerve, I was unable to detect anything but that its fibers disappear in the ganglion and cannot be traced up to any branch of the third division of the trigeminal nerve.

Furthermore, I found that positively this whole tympanic plexus can by no means be regarded—as Arnold and Beck do—as a mere ramification of the tympanic branch of the glossopharyngeal nerve. On the contrary, those are right [correct; *Gray's*, p. 1011—*ed.*] who consider the plexus as a combination of fibers of the tympanic and the lesser superficial petrosal nerve, and of sympathetic filaments belonging to the carotid plexus. It is difficult to say anything about the participation of these three nerves in the formation of the tympanic plexus and its particular branches, since the situation is different in different individuals. I believe, however, that I have found the following facts: The tympanic nerve is always the largest among those of this particular tympanic plexus; soon after having entered the tympanic cavity it sends a small branch to the round window and the mastoid air cells. It always has a part in the formation of the nerves that run toward the Eustachian tube, and finally —this seems to be of particular importance—a portion of its fibers within the lesser superficial petrosal reaches the otic ganglion and thus forms a connection between this ganglion and the [inferior] petrous ganglion of the glossopharyngeal nerve. Of course, it is hard to determine whether the strands between the otic and the inferior petrosal ganglion of IX belong to the tympanic [nerve] or to the lesser superficial petrosal, or to both. But from the thickness of the trunk of the tympanic nerve and from the branches separating from it in the tympanic cavity, I have concluded that in any case a portion of its fibers remains and forms the connection between the two ganglia.

The nerves that leave the plexus for the Eustachian tube, whose number and layout vary, are always composed of the tympanic as well as the lesser superficial petrosal nerve and certainly also—at least in some cases—of sympathetic fibers coming from the carotid; consequently, this leads to a very complicated plexus in the formation of these nerves for the Eustachian tube. Several times I definitely saw how the sympathetic fibers of the so-called lesser deep petrosal nerve passed in the shape of an arc into the nerves which run from the tympanic nerve to the Eustachian tube. On the other hand, I am not equally sure whether some of those sympathetic fibers pass into the other paths of the plexus or, vice versa, whether from the tympanic or the lesser superficial nerve certain filaments pass into the carotid canal and enter into a connection with the carotid plexus. As a whole, the course of those carotid nerves varies greatly, and I was not always able—as Arnold and others claim that they were—to detect an upper and a lower carotid ramus, or a lesser deep petrosal nerve. I must assume that this situation is caused by individual differences, since because of the type of my experiments and the study of the preparations, I feel sure that I did not overlook any small filaments, even if they were torn off.

It seemed to me that the nerve going to the oval window of the tympanic cavity belonged mainly to the lesser superficial petrosal nerve. However, I continued to have doubts about its origin, and all the more since at its origin, usually rather high up in the tympanic cavity and at the point where the lesser superficial petrosal (after its entrance into the tympanic cavity) turns at almost a right angle, I found a small microscopic ganglion.

I made this observation without knowing whether others before me had seen something similar, since in our textbooks and manuals no one has mentioned ganglia on the tympanic nerve except for Valentin (*Müller's Archiv,* 1840, p. 287, and *Nervenlehre,* p. 471), who claims to have seen a small ganglion or a ganglionic swelling on the trunk of the tympanic nerve where the latter enters the tympanic cavity through the tympanic canaliculus. Krause agrees with Valentin. I found, however, that this is an erroneous opinion, as Beck (p. 60) has already mentioned, and that at the point in question neither a ganglion nor a ganglionic enlargement exists on the trunk of the tympanic nerve. It was only later that I became acquainted with Pappenheim's *Gewebelehre des Gehororgans.* In this work I found, among a great number of amazing facts about the nerves of the tympanic cavity (p. 60), the statement that in the ox the so-called lower division of the trigeminal nerve which supposedly goes toward the membrane of the oval window has a small ganglion consisting of very few big ganglionic nodules. Furthermore, it is stated, the ganglionic enlargements are embedded in rather heavy sheaths and surrounded by nerves; the ganglion sits only superiorly; the pile of small reddish spots [we don't know what he means here. *Ed.*] which are found in other ganglia occurs here too; the ganglia are oval or round; the ramus of Jacobson's nerve going to the facial nerve contains also a greater number of ganglionic nodules than other nerves, and finally, according to Pappenheim, the trunks of all of Jacobson's nerves contain many ganglionic swellings.

Those statements are probably the source for Kölliker's remarks in his *Gewebelehre* (4th ed. p. 351): "Its [the glossopharyngeal nerve's] terminal segment contains small ganglia in the tympanic cavity and the tongue." And on page 692: "Their [the nerves of the tympanic cavity] endings are unknown; but we do know that the tympanic nerve has many big isolated ganglion cells that lie together in small nodules."

I agree with these findings only in that I have usually found—as mentioned above—in the nerve for the oval window a small ganglion, and once I found one in the path of the greater superficial petrosal nerve. At least in humans the other nerves of this tympanic plexus never have ganglia. It seems strange that Pappenheim claims to have seen ganglia on the ramus of Jacobson's nerve going to the facial nerve while, as I shall show further down, such a ramus does not exist.

Finally, I wish to talk about the small connecting strand observed by many authors between the genu of the facial nerve and the lesser superficial petrosal nerve at the point where the latter descends into the tympanic cavity. After many experiments concerning this particular point I must agree with Beck. Between the greater and lesser superficial petrosal nerve there exists a small artery and vein, which at the point where the superficial petrosal turns to descend into the tympanic cavity is split with minor variations into several small branches, of which one usually descends together with the lesser superficial petrosal into the tympanic cavity, while another runs toward the genu of the facial nerve and continues close to the periphery of that nerve. This situation can easily give the illusion of an anastomosis between the genu of the facial and the lesser superficial petrosal nerve. However, not only the microscopic analysis of these apparent twigs themselves, but also the meticulous examination of the entire genu of the facial nerve and the relevant location of the lesser superficial petrosal show that no nerve filaments exist anywhere in this area. I believe that this wrong opinion must be eliminated from anatomical findings, and that Longet's theory about the motor root of the otic ganglion should not be derived from it. Incidentally, Arnold has already expressed his doubts about the existence of such an anastomosis (*Anatomie,* II, pp. 868, 910).

VI. The Vagus and the Spinal Accessory Nerve of Willis

Although the vagus nerve is spread out over a wide area, and although its branches have numerous connections with spinal and sympathetic nerves, it has only few important anastomoses with other cranial nerves which would fall into the realm of my study. After its exit from the jugular foramen it is connected through short strands with its neighbors, the glossopharyngeal, the spinal accessory of Willis, and the hypoglossal nerve. I have already mentioned the first one as well as the interesting auricular branch of the vagus and its connection with the facial nerve [Figures 71-77]. Therefore, I will now turn at once to the accessory nerve which is closely connected with it and for that reason was previously regarded as part of it.

It has been known for a long time that during its passage in the vertebral canal the spinal accessory is sometimes connected with the posterior roots of the second and more often the first cervical nerve; about thirty years ago this fact became of particular importance because of Scarpa's, Arnold's, and Th. L. W. Bischoff's theory of the purely motor nature of the accessory nerve, which led to a manifold meticulous study. J. C. Mayer (*Acta nat. Curios.*, V, XVI, P. II, pp. 784, 1833) described eight different origins of the posterior root of the first cervical nerve and their connections with the accessory nerve; in one of those the posterior root was missing entirely, and only further up a thread of the accessory replaced the root by passing from the back through the first intervertebral foramen. J. Müller described a similar case (*Archiv für Anat.*, 1824, p. 12). The same authors, as well as Hyrtl (*Med. Jahrb. d. osterr. Monarchie,* Neueste Folge, Bd. X, p. 445) spoke of small ganglia which appear at the roots or even at the trunk of the accessory nerve, and they expressed their belief that this fact was contradictory to its purely motor nature. Even before these observations had been published, however, Bischoff in his *Commentatio de Nervi Accessori. Anat. et Phys.*, p. 12, 1832 had mentioned that those connections of the posterior root of the first cervical nerve with the accessory nerve are not genuine, inasmuch as the fibers, although they are extremely close to the accessory

FIGURE 71

This figure shows the trunks of the glossopharyngeal, the vagus, the spinal accessory nerve of Willis, and the hypoglossal nerve and their connections with each other.

a glossopharyngeal nerve

b vagus nerve

c spinal accessory of Willis

d hypoglossal nerve

e apparent anastomosis between vagus and hypoglossal nerve, after the latter has been rendered visible by turning its lower end sideways

f f' f'' anastomosis between glossopharyngeal nerve and vagus

g origin of the auricular branch of the vagus where a bundle running peripherally can be seen

h tympanic nerve

i first cervical nerve and its connection with the hypoglossal nerve

k sympathetic thread to the hypoglossal nerve

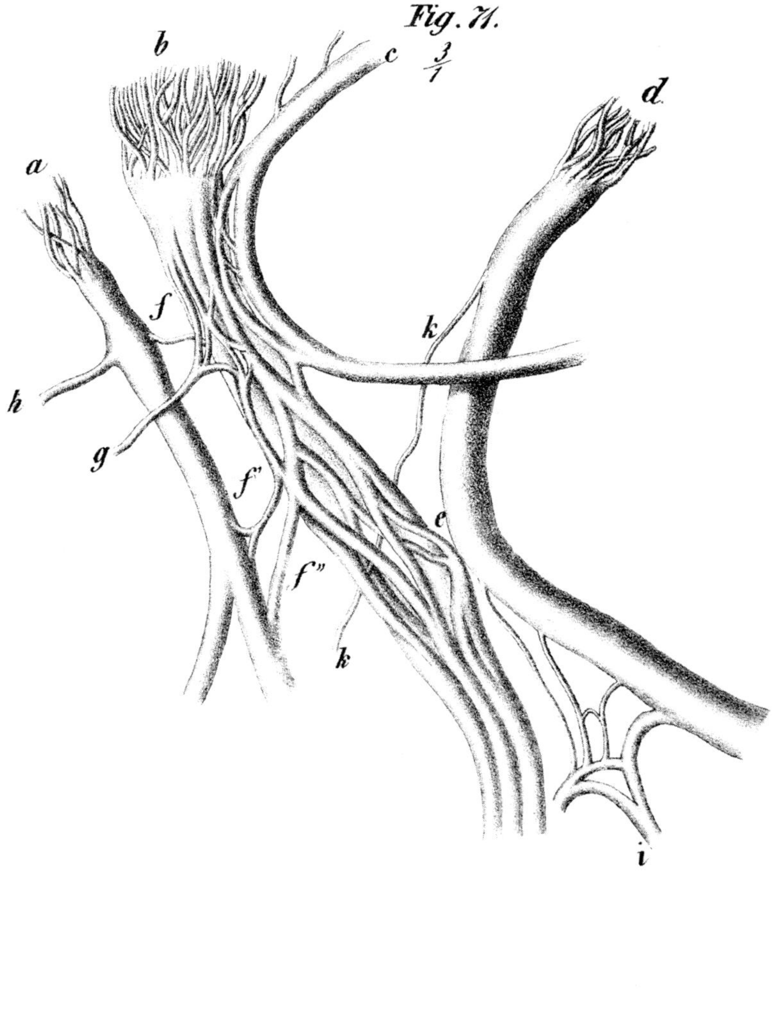

FIGURES 72 TO 77

These figures show the connection between vagus and spinal accessory, as they leave the jugular foramen.

Figures 72 and 73, 74 and 75, and 76 and 77 belong together, as in each case the particular items are shown from the front and from the back. It is difficult to determine the boundary between the roots of both nerves.

a vagus

b spinal accessory

c inner branch of (b) going to (a)

It can be seen everywhere that before the inner branch is given up to the vagus, there are connections between the two nerves which can be regarded as bundles of the vagus going to the spinal accessory; but they could also be roots of the spinal accessory involved in the formation of the jugular ganglion of the vagus nerve.

Fig. 72. $\frac{3}{1}$

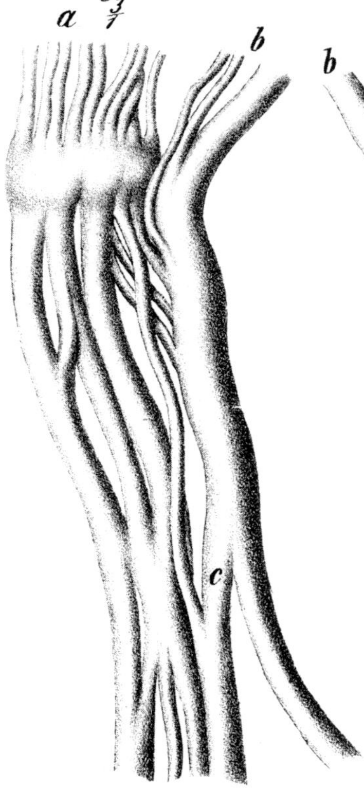

Fig. 73. $\frac{3}{1}$

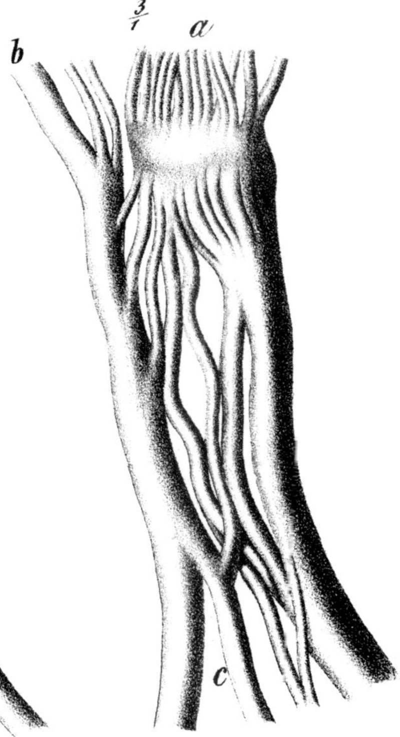

Fig. 74.

4/1

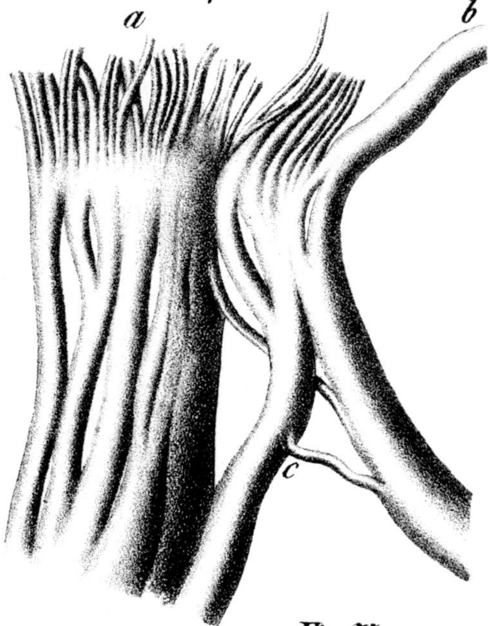

Fig. 76.

3/1

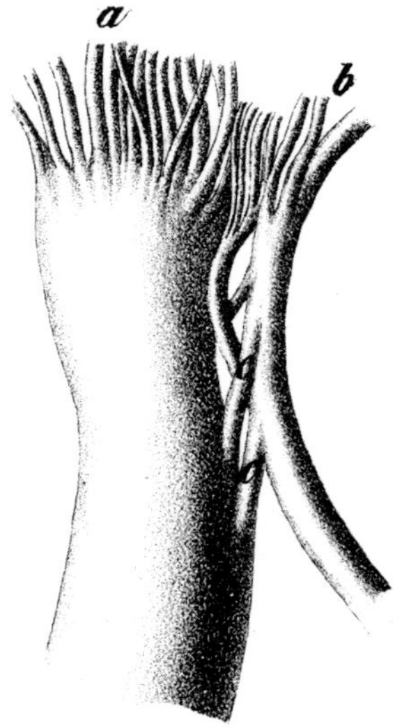

Fig. 75.

4/1

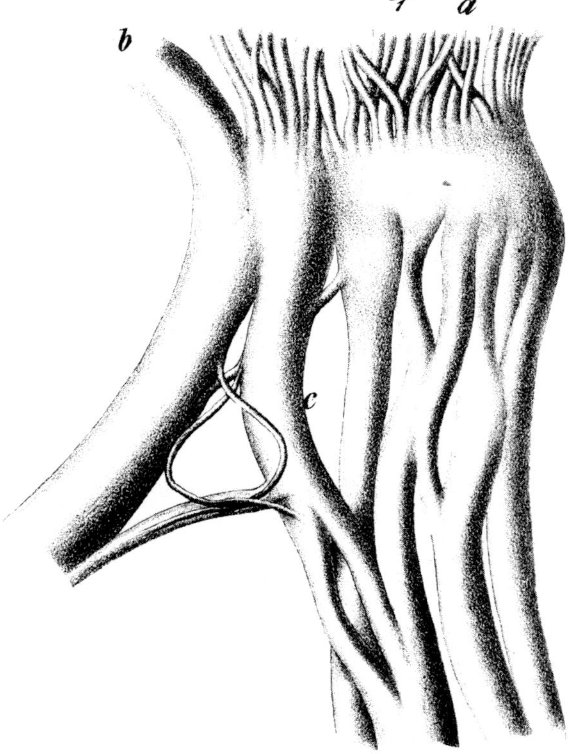

Fig. 77.

3/1

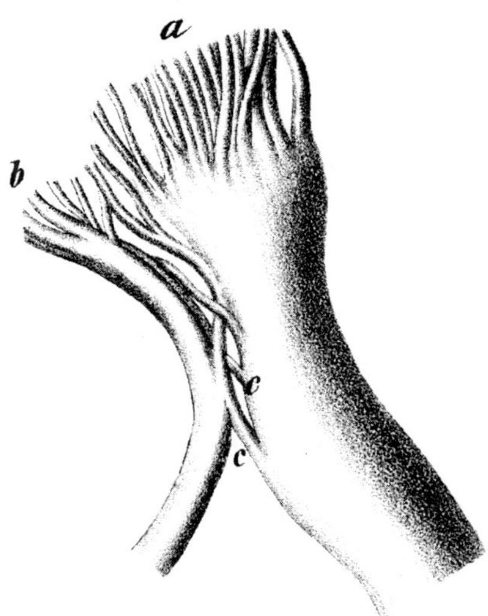

and even enter its sheath, leave it again and run to the anterior root. Arnold agreed with this opinion (*Tiedemann's Zeitschrift,* V, p. 177, "Bemerkungen über das Hirn," p. 182) and he never changed his mind. If a ganglion is found at a root connected with the accessory nerve or at the latter's trunk, it belongs to the posterior root which in those cases lies within the dura meter.

In the "Jahresbericht für 1836," *Archiv* 1837, p. 279, Müller had described his case in a way that could hardly be called sufficient as an explanation for the anastomosis involved. Not only was the posterior root of the first cervical nerve missing and was further up—supplied with a small ganglion—separated from the accessory nerve, but after an exact analysis of the separation of this root from the trunk of the accessory, Müller became convinced that the root consisted of two fascicles, one ascending from below and one descending from above from the trunk of the accessory nerve. Furthermore, he saw that the uppermost root of the accessory, which originates above the posterior end of the olive at its entrance into the brain stem, is also divided into two fascicles, one ascending and one descending; therefore, he assumed—probably rightly—that the descending fascicle was the posterior root of the first cervical nerve. Consequently, the latter was formed in a very strange way by roots of the accessory nerve [Figures 78-87].

A meticulous analysis of the point in question which was repeated several times proved that the earlier findings were correct. But I also discovered a few facts that have never before been described. I saw that the relation of the posterior root of the first cervical nerve to the accessory varies greatly. I shall mention only a few of the cases that are similar to Müller's observation and could only be explained in the same manner.

Although in one case a posterior root of the first cervical nerve existed, left the dura mater in back of the ascending accessory together with the vertebral artery, formed its ganglion in the intervertebral foramen, and merged with the anterior root, yet one of the strands of this posterior root—while still within the dura mater—received a supporting strand from the upper end of the trunk of the accessory nerve, and therefore it seemed that its fibers ran peripherally at both ends. I do not doubt that this seemingly impossible situation could be explained by the possibility that from a root of the accessory, located at a still higher point, fibers ran backward peripherally into the trunk of the accessory then left it and passed peripherally into the one strand of the posterior root; but I was not able to verify this assumption, since the preparation had already been cut out.

In a second case the posterior root of the first cervical nerve was totally missing at its usual place of origin, just as in Müller's case.

FIGURES 78 TO 87

These figures give pictures of the varying connection between the spinal accessory nerve of Willis and the posterior root of the first cervical nerve.

a peripheral end of the spinal accessory

b anterior root of first cervical nerve

c posterior root of the first cervical nerve

d ganglion of the posterior root of the first cervical nerve

e false ganglia

f posterior root of the second cervical nerve

Fig. 78. 3/1

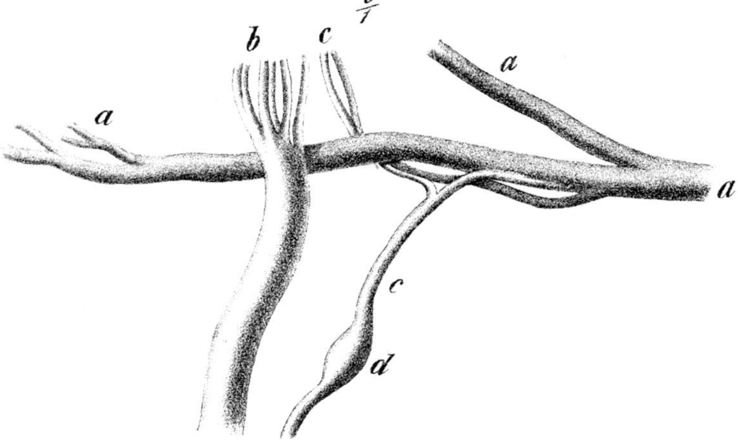

Fig. 79. 3/1

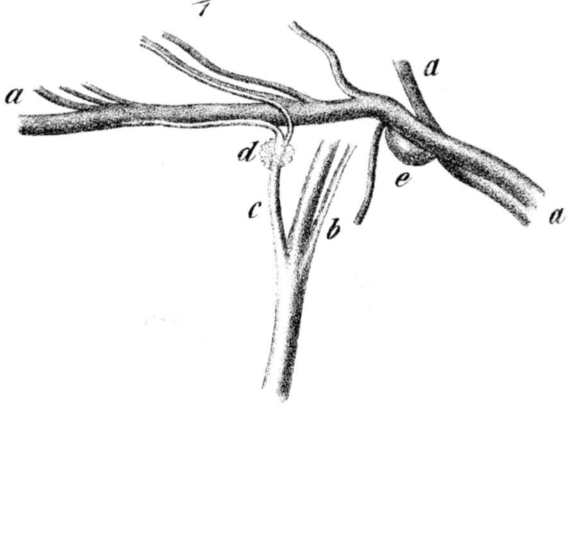

Fig. 80.

3/1

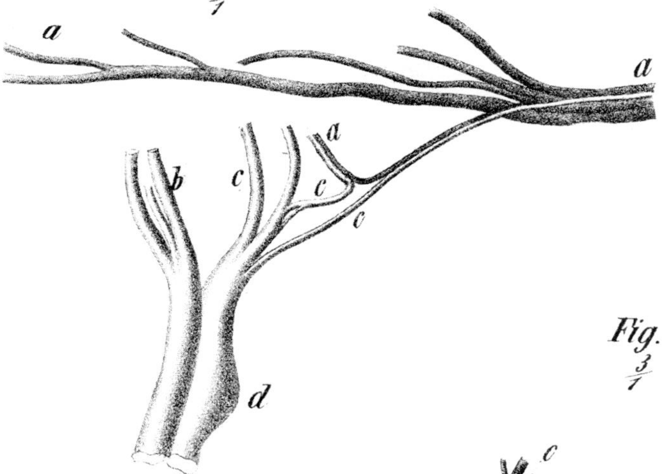

Fig. 81.

3/1

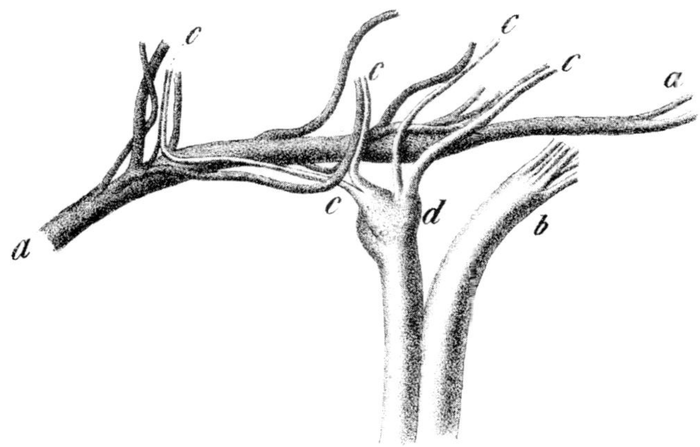

Fig. 82.

3/1

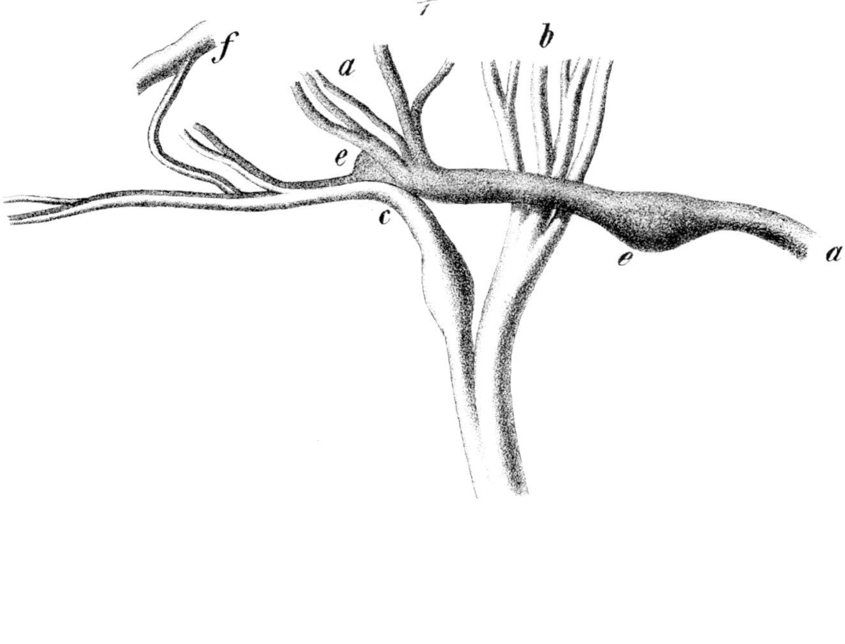

Fig. 83.
3/1

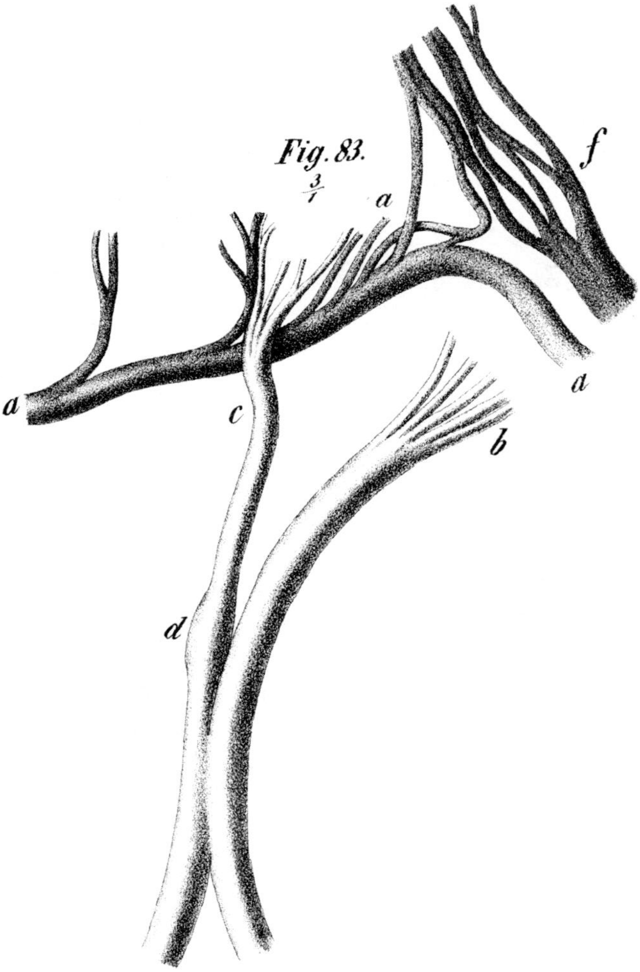

Fig. 84.
3/1

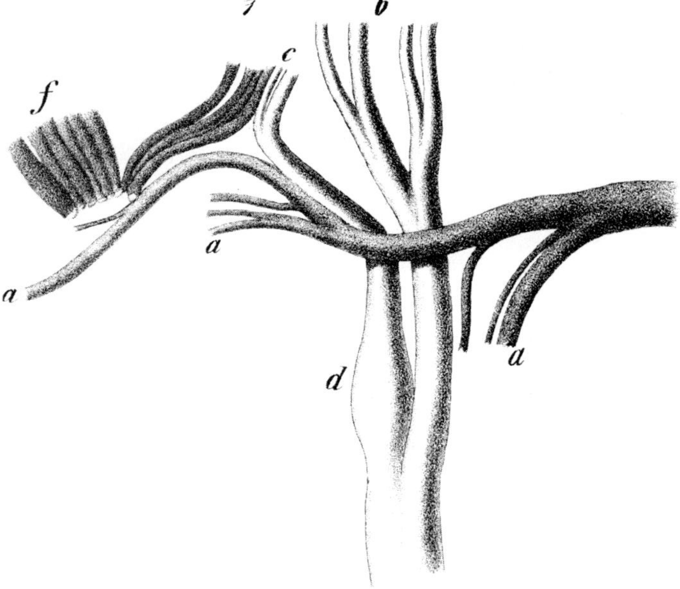

Fig. 85.
3/1

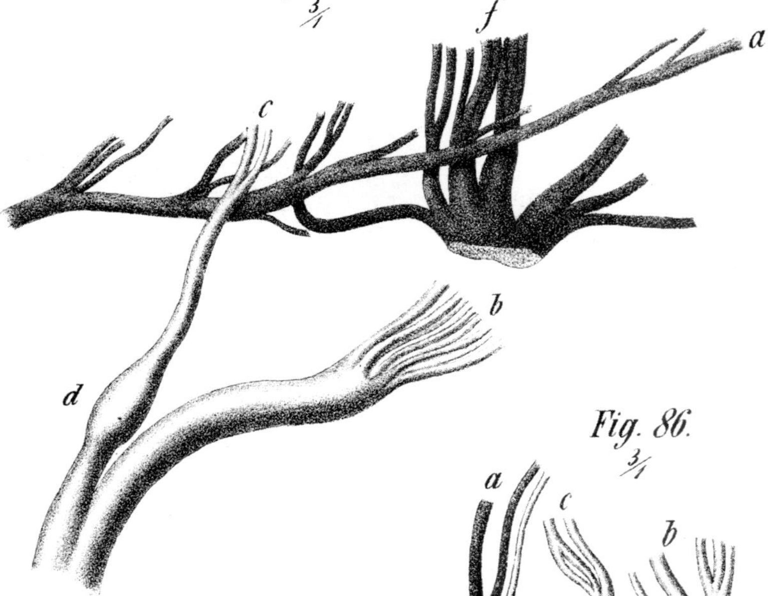

Fig. 86.
3/1

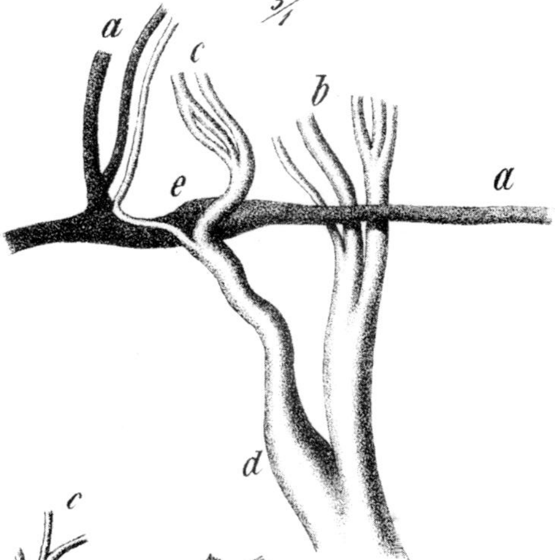

Fig. 87.
3/1

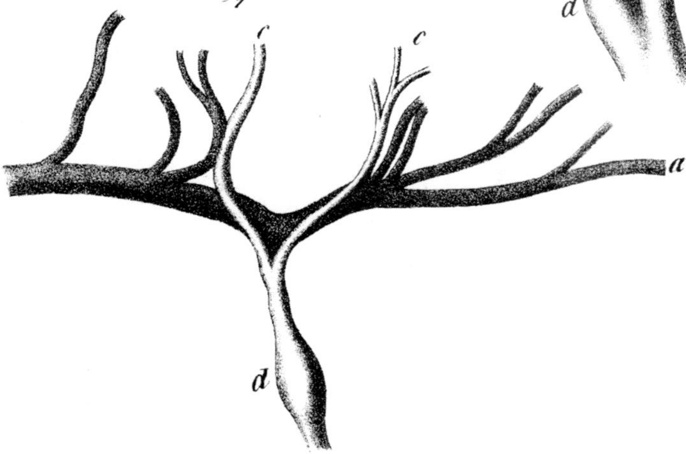

But at a higher point a strand left the accessory nerve, turned downward, went close to the vertebral artery where it had a small ganglion, then left the dura mater and merged with the anterior rather strong root, thus substituting for the posterior root. But the manner of the rootlets coming into being was peculiar. For—as with Müller's—it grew out of two fascicles, one that originated from a higher root of the accessory and a second one that descended peripherally from the trunk of this nerve. Unquestionably, the latter fascicle originated from a root that passed into the trunk of the accessory, from which a group ran backward into the trunk of the accessory and then entered the posterior root of the first cervical nerve.

I shall now present the story of a third very strange case. At first sight it seemed that a sizable posterior root of the first cervical nerve closely approached the trunk of the accessory; at its closest point it had a greyish-reddish ganglion, crossed the accessory, and left the dura mater together with the vertebral artery and finally merged with the anterior root, after having formed another ganglion. At a higher spot on the side of the accessory, where it was not connected with any root, there was a third greyish-reddish ganglion. But when I studied the connection and the exit of the posterior root of the cervical nerve across the trunk of the accessory under the magnifying glass, I found to my amazement that without any doubt these roots did *not* pass into the real root, but ascended into the trunk of the accessory, and that at the same location the major portion of the trunk of the accessory, which was composed of the lower root strands, merged with the posterior root of the first cervical nerve. On the other hand, I could not see whether the two small ganglia within the dura mater really contained ganglionic enlargements; nor did I detect nerves going through them. They consisted solely of a fine granular, rather smooth substance easily detachable from the nerve. In former times such formations were surely regarded as genuine ganglia, particularly by Hyrtl, but only the ganglia outside the dura mater contained real ganglionic nodules with a slight pigmentation.

In still another case the first cervical nerve started with an unusually strong posterior root, which came close alongside the trunk of the accessory nerve but seemed to bypass it; it left the dura mater together with the vertebral artery, formed its ganglion, and merged with the anterior root. However, a close examination showed that at the point where the trunk of the accessory joined the posterior root, a strand of the latter joined the accessory and continued its course peripherally without ever leaving it. The same was true of a strand of the posterior root of the second cervical nerve.

Still another case was remarkable, because the posterior root of the first cervical nerve was not only very closely connected with the trunk of the accessory, although it did leave it later, but one of the branches of this posterior root descended to the posterior root of the second cervical nerve and left the dura mater with it.

I saw still more variations of arrangements and connections of the posterior aspect of the first cervical nerve, which I will discuss later, together with the description of the figures. From what has been said so far, the definite conclusion can be drawn that there is no strict division between the posterior roots and the trunk of the accessory nerve. The latter participates in the formation of the former and, as far as can be determined, the former participates in the formation of the trunk of the accessory, although at the end they follow again their separate courses. Both kinds of roots have the same origin from the spinal cord, and therefore it cannot be denied that the accessory nerve possesses sensory fibers among its roots.

A second connection of the accessory nerve occurs with the vagus during the passage through the foramen lacerum [jugular]. Regarding this connection, the doctrine of Scarpa, Arnold, and Bischoff has been almost completely verified, namely that the accessory passes the (inferior)* jugular ganglion of the vagus nerve located in the foramen lacerum† jugular without having a close contact with it, then is divided into an inner and an outer branch, of which the former joins the vagus and partially merges with the pharyngeal ramus, while the latter is destined for the sternocleidomastoid and the trapezius muscles.

In spite of a careful study I find it quite hard to analyze that particular spot. It is extremely difficult to determine which of the roots are the uppermost ones of the accessory and which ones are the lowest of the vagus, and of course this makes it very hard to establish whether the roots of the accessory participate in the jugular ganglion. The problem could be solved by claiming that all roots that pass into the [jugular] ganglion belong to the vagus, and those that bypass them go to the accessory. However, this does not lead to a solution either, for immediately behind the [jugular] ganglion the connections begin between the ganglion and the accessory, which is consequently separated. Among them there usually exists a group which goes from the [jugular] ganglion to the accessory; it seems to me therefore that the question cannot be answered

*[True according to *Gray's Anatomy*, 1973, but still, strangely, a matter of argument. *Ed.*]

†[This is obviously an error! Bischoff shows in the next paragraph that he, of course, knew that the accessory and vagus go through the jugular foramen. *Ed.*]

in the foregoing manner. Since, however, Lobstein, Martin, Boyer, and Bischoff have observed—the first three in humans and Bischoff in the calf—that the accessory nerve enters the *jugular foramen* through a special opening and sheath of the dura mater; separated from the vagus and its jugular ganglion, it may be concluded that the accessory does not take part in the formation of this ganglion, not even with some of its roots. This, in turn, leads to the conclusion that—as Spencer has claimed (*Edinb. Med. and Surg. Journal,* 1842, p. 397)—a root of the vagus always bypasses the ganglion and merges with the accessory.

My studies of the connection of the accessory with the vagus nerve at the far side of the ganglion have shown that it is never as simple as it has usually been described, namely that the accessory is merely divided into two branches, of which the innermost merges with the vagus, while the outermost continues its course toward the muscles. In contrast, after having brightened the very firm connection of the accessory with the vagus with acetic acid, and by using compression, I have always found that a multiple exchange of nerve fibers exists between the vagus and the accessory, whereby the accessory usually furnishes fibers to the vagus, although sometimes it also happens the other way around. As is well known, fibers that originate from the accessory usually merge with the pharyngeal ramus of the vagus nerve.

Volkmann (*Müller's Archiv,* 1844, p. 511) has described an anastomosis of the outermost branch of the accessory with the second and third cervical nerve. Strangely enough, this observation has remained completely unnoticed, although it points out one of those loops without end. Volkmann describes these anastomoses mainly as occurring in the calf, but he claims that he has also seen them in men, horses, dogs, and cats; he has even made experiments on living animals and believes that it is chiefly through these anastomoses that sensory fibers are furnished to the accessory. This anastomosis occurs within the fibers of the sternocleidomastoid muscle, while the accessory nerve is passing through it. From what I have seen, this connection is always formed by a branch of the third cervical nerve [Figures 88-91], which it usually leaves together with the nerve which is to form an anastomosis with the descending ramus of the hypoglossal nerve; soon, however, it separates from the latter. Often the ansa of the second cervical nerve approaches at a short distance the point where it leaves the third branch, which fact might lead to the conclusion that this too contributes to the anastomosis; but that is not the case. The aforementioned branch of the third cervical nerve then runs in the shape of a downward pointing convex arc among the branches of the posterior edge of the sternocleidomastoid and thus approaches the trunk of the accessory at such a close distance that it looks like a simple anastomosis between the two. However, this is by no means true. Before reaching the accessory nerve, the third cervical nerve has split into two branches, which lie close together. When they reach the trunk of the accessory, one of those branches crosses the accessory, continues into the sternocleidomastoid, meets the ramifications of the branch which has already left the accessory at a higher point and whose destination is this muscle, and finally [C3] enters the muscle together with the more delicate ramifications of the latter [XI], and forms a second more delicate anastomosis. The other portion of the [third] cervical nerve is soon divided into various branches, ascends along the trunk of the accessory, which at this point is usually divided into several bundles and forms a plexus with them. It is very difficult and sometimes impossible to follow the path of the fibers through the plexus. I believe, however, that finer threads of this ramus of the accessory as well as the ramus of the [third] cervical nerve run in a straight line, form a loop-shaped anastomosis with finer branches of the accessory, and according to Volkmann's and Hyrtl's concept, this anastomosis seems to be without an end. Yet the path centrally is too long and too complicated and therefore the opinion cannot be verified, for there is no lack of opportunities for a separation of the fibers that seem to run in a central direction. It seems that Volkmann has studied this anastomosis only in the calf. In humans the situation is certainly not as simple as it sounds according to his description, and the anastomosis can only be detected by fine filaments made visible under the magnifying glass. It is very difficult to analyze the aforementioned plexus, and I had the impression that it also contains sympathetic fibers.

FIGURES 88 TO 91

They depict the anastomosis between the spinal accessory of Willis and the third cervical nerve among the bundles of the sternocleidomastoid muscle.

Figures 89, 90, and 91 seem to show an anastomosis without end.

a spinal accessory of Willis

b ramus sternocleidomastoid of (a)

c second cervical nerve, which is not involved in the anastomosis

d third cervical nerve, which with its branch

e forms the anastomosis with (b) with its branch

f forms an anastomosis situated further down with the trunk of the accessory

Fig. 88.
3/1

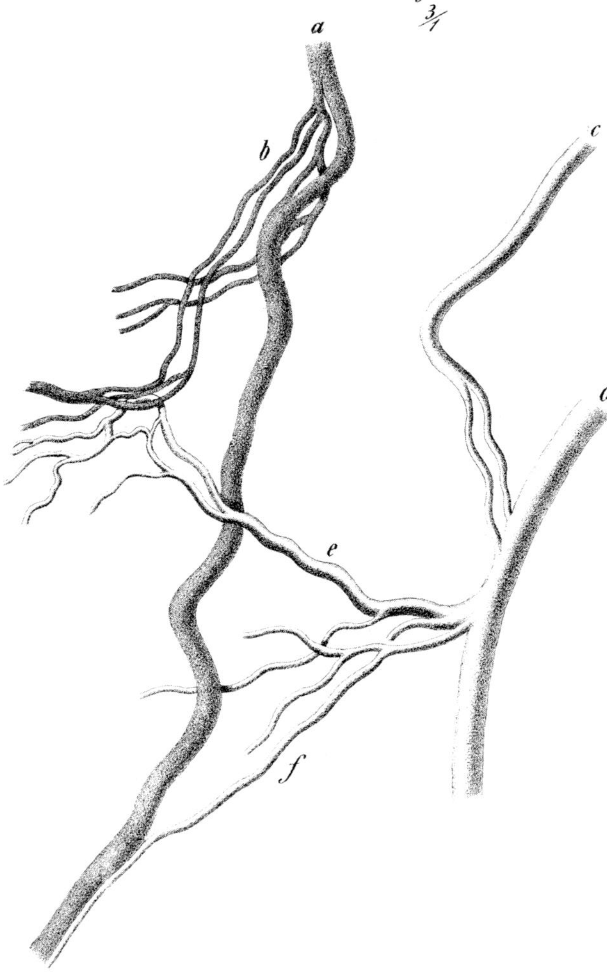

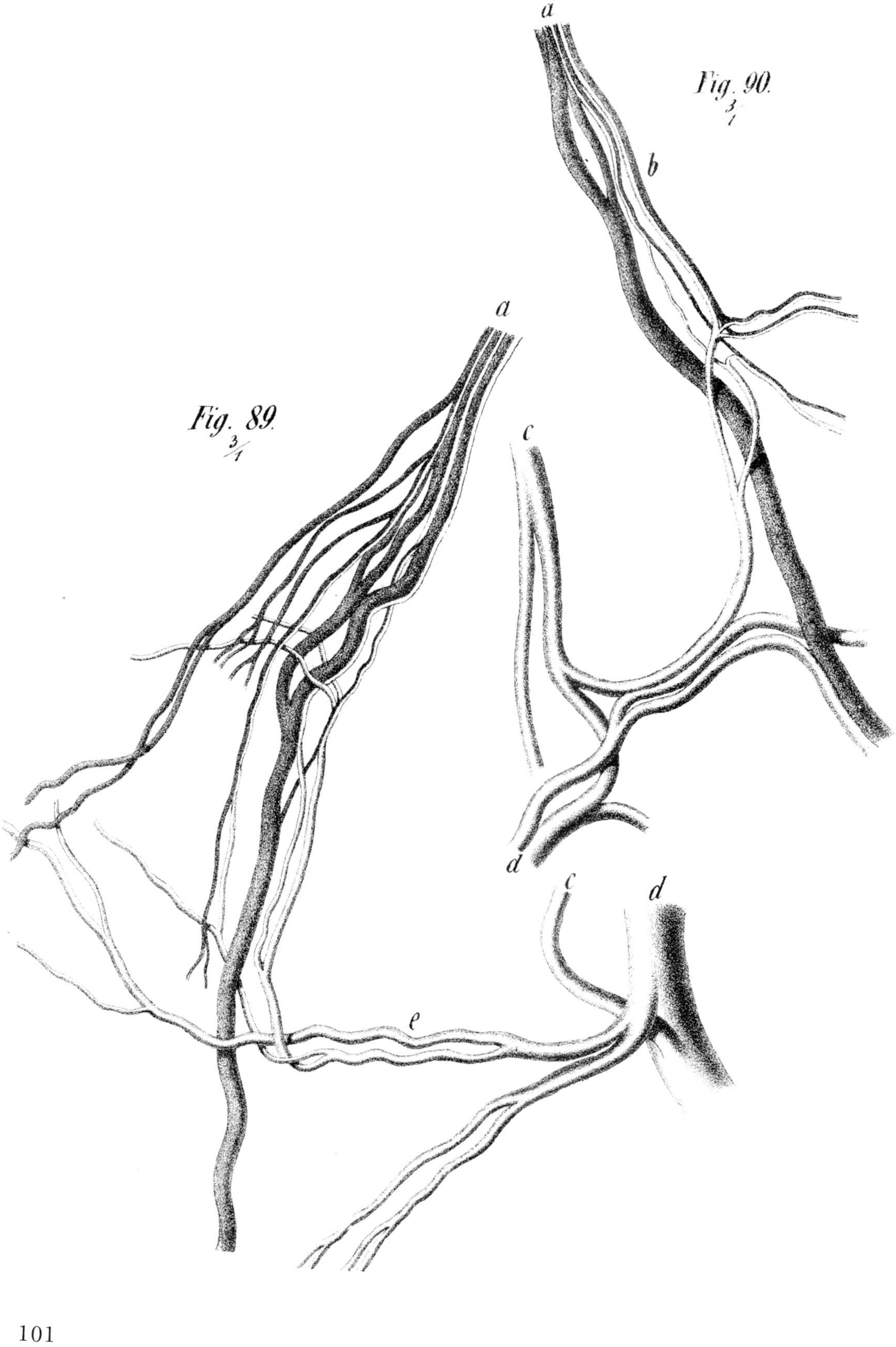

Fig. 90. 3/1

Fig. 89. 3/1

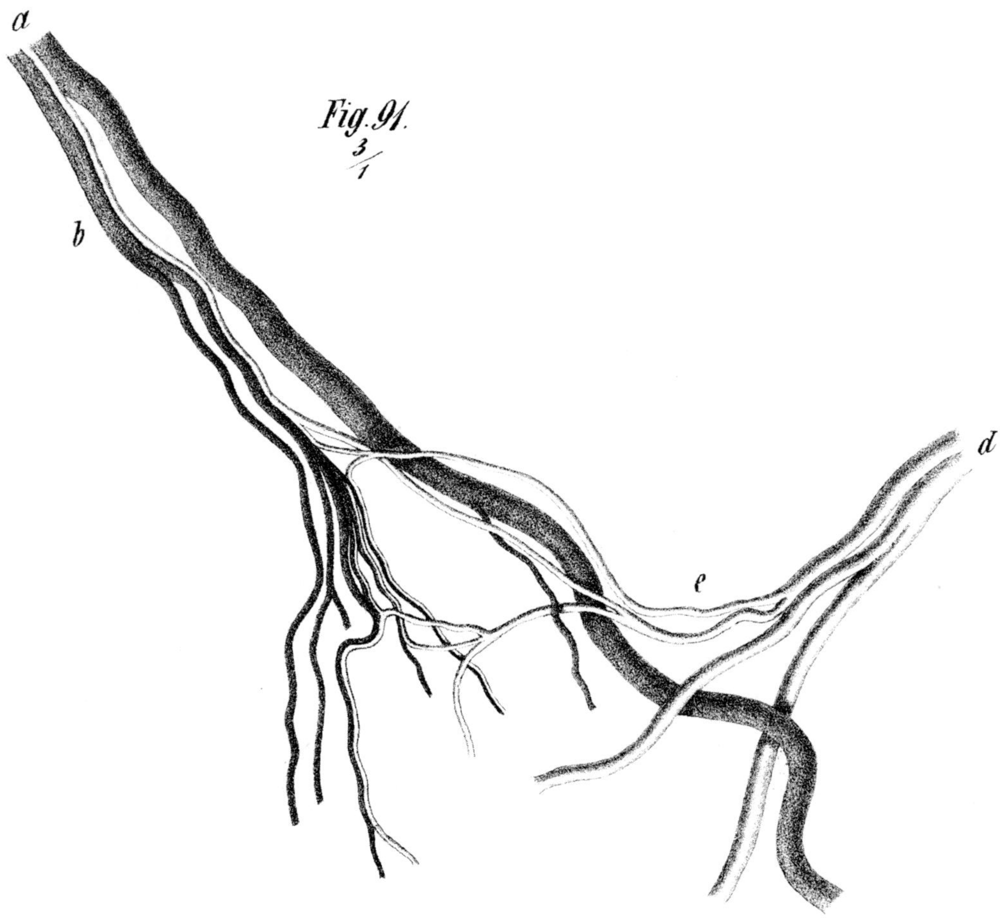
a
Fig. 91.
3/1
b
d
e

VII. The Hypoglossal Nerve

It has been generally accepted that the hypoglossal nerve passes through the anterior condyloid foramen, runs close to the trunk of the vagus, and after crossing diagonally over the latter turns downward and inward. At this point it joins the first and the second cervical nerve and usually also the vagus.

Since according to Hyrtl (*Nat. Hist. Review,* Jan. 1863, p. 95) the connection with the first cervical nerve belongs to the nerve loops without end, I have paid particular attention to the latter, whereby I met with greater difficulties than I had expected. Sappey (p. 305) says that there are usually two branches, of which one merges with the first cervical ansa, while the other one descends along the trunk of the hypoglossal nerve and, at least partially, merges with the descending ramus of the latter. The first branch is probably the one which Hyrtl calls the loop without end. I myself have found this connection with the first cervical nerve to be sometimes stronger, sometimes weaker, sometimes brought about by one and sometimes by several threads.

I always detected a very fine nerve which seemed to leave the anterior branch of the first cervical nerve at the point where the latter is divided into its several branches. This ascended up to the condyloid foramen along the trunk of the hypoglossal nerve with which it merged; or the direction could have been the other way around, namely from the hypoglossal nerve into the first cervical nerve. That would have been a loop without end. However, after extensive studies I am convinced that, in spite of all appearances, those strands originate not from the first cervical nerve but from sympathetic fibers, which form with the branches of the first ramus, a very complicated and hard-to-untangle plexus. Perhaps this nerve belongs to those that according to Luschka and Rudiger penetrate the condyloid foramen into the cranial cavity and spread out in the dura mater and its sinus. But there can be no doubt that it merged with the hypoglossal nerve [Figures 92-96].

Furthermore, I saw sometimes, although not always, how a branch passed from the first cervical nerve centrally into the trunk of the hypoglossal nerve; this would constitute a loop without end,

FIGURES 92 TO 96

They show several connecting strands between the hypoglossal and the vagus nerve—Figures 92 and 94 form the latter to the former and Figure 93 forms the former to the latter.

a hypoglossal nerve

b vagus nerve

cc connecting strands going from vagus to hypoglossal and vice versa

d first cervical nerve and its connections with the hypoglossal nerve

e in Figure 94 an apparent anastomosis between vagus and hypoglossal nerves

Figure 95. Connection of the first cervical nerve (d) with the hypoglossal nerve (a).
At (f) a connection between the pharyngeal ramus of the vagus and the pharyngeal ramus of the glossopharyngeal (e).

Figure 96. Connections of the first cervical nerve with the hypoglossal nerve, some of which pass centrally and others peripherally into the hypoglossal nerve.

g sympathetic nerve going to the hypoglossal nerve

Fig. 92.

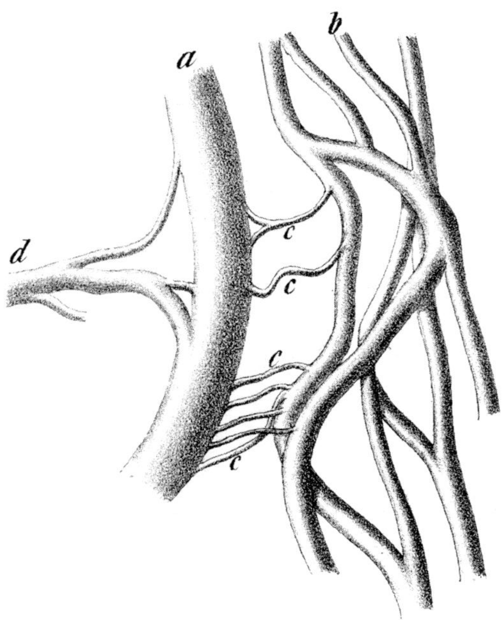

Fig. 93.

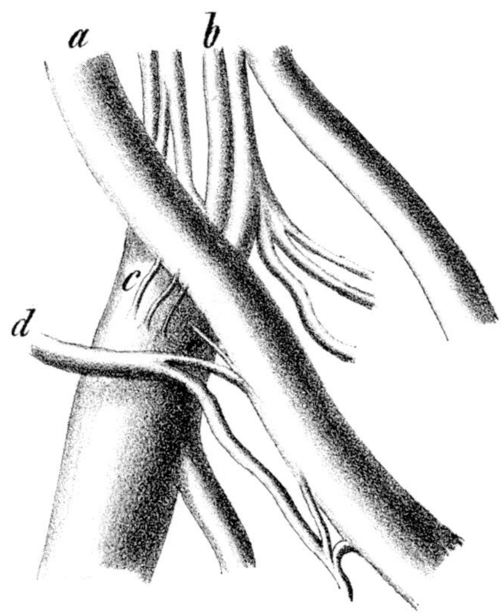

Fig. 95.

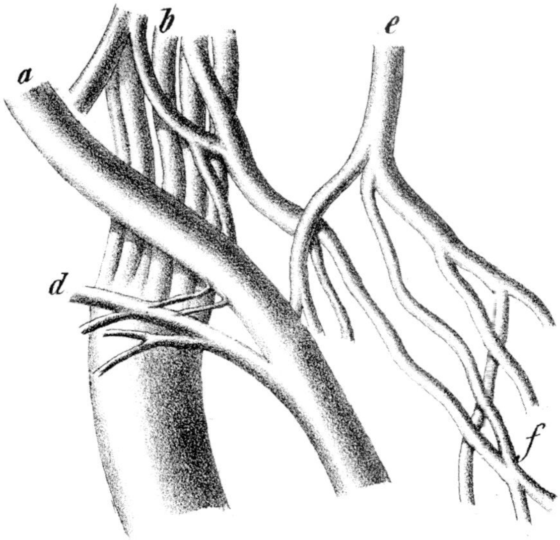

Fig. 94.

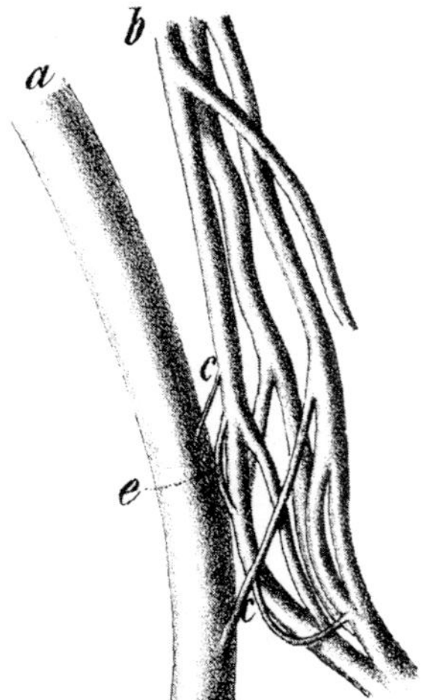

Fig. 96.

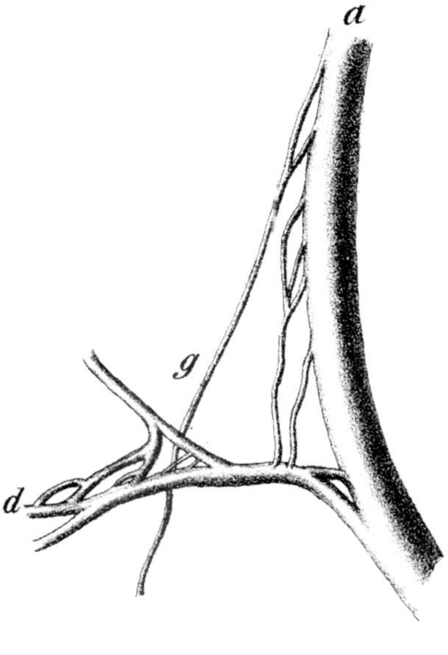

unless one would assume that it runs from the hypoglossal nerve to the first cervical nerve and spreads out in one of the branches of the latter. But I could not detect any such course of a branch of the first cervical nerve.

In addition, it seems that there are always one or more branches of the first cervical nerve, which merge peripherally with the trunk of the hypoglossal nerve. In that case, one can indeed observe how sometimes the strongest of those branches descends at the outer edge of the hypoglossal nerve in such a manner that it is possible to trace it at least partially to the descending ramus of the latter, although on the way it also forms a plexus with other fibers of the hypoglossal nerve. Such a course is by no means the rule, however, and often after the connection of the cervical branch with the hypoglossal nerve has taken place, it is not possible to say anything about the further course of the fibers.

All existing manuals state that the hypoglossal nerve joins the vagus and particularly its ganglioform plexus through one or more twigs at the point where it crosses above the latter. Almost no one, however, describes details of this connection. Valentin (p. 518) even distinguishes between an upper and a lower connection, and he apparently believes that the strands of both connections go from the hypoglossal to the vagus nerve. Longet (p. 409) and Sappey (p. 305) agree with Valentin. On the other hand, Boehmer ("De nono pari nervi cerebri" in Ludwig's *Script. neurol.,* I, p. 294) denies that those connecting strands exist, and he is of the opinion that strands of connective tissues had been mistaken for them.

My own point of view lies somewhere midway between the two opinions. No doubt several very fine and short connecting fascicles usually exist between the hypoglossal and the vagus nerve at the spot where the former crosses the latter. As far as I could make out, however, those strands went from the vagus to the hypoglossal nerve and not the other way around. I am just as certain that those thicker fibers usually described as going from the hypoglossal to the vagus nerve in reality are not a connection between the two nerves. It is true that in general two rather thick fibers of the vagus run so closely alongside the hypoglossal nerve that anyone who has not made a meticulous study of this particular place and has not first swabbed it with acetic acid will assume that they are connecting branches. But having made an exact exploration with the use of acetic acid I saw under the magnifying glass that those strands really do not merge with the hypoglossal nerve, but join the rest of the fibers of the ganglioform plexus of the vagus nerve. However, I do not deny that occasionally a thicker branch of the vagus merges with the hypoglossal nerve and participates, it seems to me, in the formation of the descending ramus of the latter [Figures 97-98].

Volkmann was the first to give a rather detailed description of the descending ramus of the hypoglossal nerve, after it had been known for quite some time that it is composed of strands of the hypoglossal, the vagus, the sympathetic, and in particular the cervical nerves (*Müller's Archiv,* 1840, pp. 501, 512). According to Volkmann this ramus belongs to the cranial nerves rather than to the hypoglossal. He stated that fibers of the cervical nerves go upward and run peripherally in the trunk of the hypoglossal; he had recognized this by means of an anatomical study of the point of origin of the descending ramus as well as by way of experiments which enabled him to cause twitchings in the glossal muscles of freshly killed animals by stimulating the cervical nerves. Furthermore, he believed he could prove that endloops of nerve bundles lie in the connection of the cranial nerves with the hypoglossal nerve through the descending ramus; these endloops must therefore run either from the medulla oblongata through the hypoglossal and its descending ramus and through the cervical nerves back to the spinal cord, or vice versa from the cervical cord through the cervical nerves through the descending ramus and the hypoglossal nerve to the medulla oblongata, thus forming a so-called retrograde anastomosis. Volkmann claimed that on the one hand he had discovered —particularly in the sheep—that a much greater number of fibers run from the hypoglossal nerve into the descending ramus than the latter contains below the connection with the cervical nerve—provided the number of fibers of the latter going to the descending ramus are disregarded. It could be concluded from the foregoing facts that the major portion of fibers which run from the hypoglossal nerve into the descending ramus do not remain there but return through the cervical nerve to the spinal cord (Volkmann, p. 513). On the other hand, he also discovered that when the hypoglossal nerve of animals was stimulated, the cervical nerves twitched only very rarely and among those only the sternothyroid, while as mentioned earlier this phenomenon did occur when the cervical nerves were stimulated (Volkmann, p. 502).

Valentin, without mentioning those statements by Volkmann, says in his *Hirn und Nervenlehre,* 1841, p. 520, in an annotation: "A plexus always occurs at the spot where the descending ramus originates from the hypoglossal nerve, and branches from the trunk of the hypoglossal nerve definitely enter here; this can clearly be seen through exact examinations. Consequently, the descending ramus is not just a product of the cervical nerves." Arnold in his *Handbuch der Anatomie,* II, p. 838, 1851, notes also, without mentioning Volkmann, that the cervical ramus of the hypoglossal nerve is a mixture of fibers of this nerve, the vagus, and the cervical nerves. Central arc-shaped fibers run inside the ansa; but whether

FIGURES 97 TO 98

Two preparations of the connection between hypoglossal and vagus nerves. Figure 97 is seen somewhat higher from the front, Figure 98 somewhat lower from the rear.

a glossopharyngeal nerve

b vagus nerve

c hypoglossal nerve

Figure 97 shows a strong strand going from the vagus to the hypoglossal nerve, and Figure 98 shows at (e) a slightly thinner strand going from the hypoglossal nerve to the vagus. In addition, Figure 97 shows in (f) the anastomosis between the pharyngeal ramus of the glossopharyngeal nerve and the pharyngeal ramus of the vagus nerve.

Fig. 97.

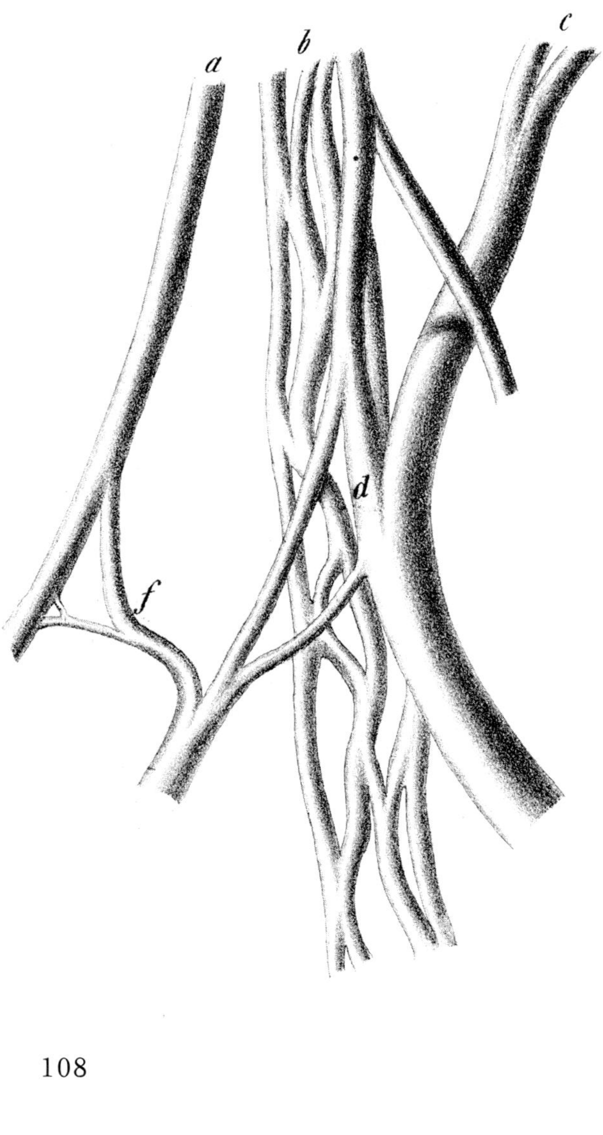

Fig. 98.

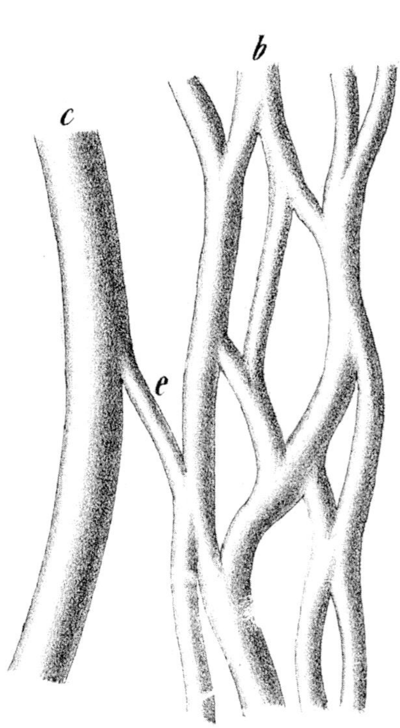

they belong to the twelfth cranial nerve or to the second and third cervical nerves or to both cannot be stated with certainty.

Longet, who does not mention Volkmann either, says in his *Anatomie und Physiologie des Nervensystems* (1842, II, p. 411) that according to its origin the descending ramus belongs to the cervical nerves as much as it does or perhaps even more than to the hypoglossal nerve. He came to this conclusion by assuming that it originates from fibers of the two upper cervical nerves, which join the hypoglossal nerve above the point where the descending ramus begins. He claims that it merges in the shape of a loop with the inner-descending branch of the cervical plexus, and that it supplies from the curve of this arc several cervical nerves with a number of branches. Longet did not undertake any experiments in regard to the function of those nerves. Sappey (*Anat. descriptive,* 1852, II, p. 306) states that the descending ramus leaves the hypoglossal nerve in two groups of which one leaves the trunk at the center, while the other one enters it at the periphery. After that, he claims, it connects in a plexiform ansa with a trunk composed of the third and fourth cervical nerves. Longet continues saying that the latter is divided into two branches, of which the lower one joins the descending ramus and forms together with it a small plexus, from which the nerves for the cervical muscles originate. The upper one proceeds next to the descending ramus, returns alongside the latter, and enters the hypoglossal nerve peripherally. For the study of this situation he used a concentrated solution of potassium and aluminum sulfate. Again Volkmann, who had already earlier recognized the same facts, is not mentioned. Sappey did not accept Volkmann's theory of the endloops in the anastomosis (see No. 1, p. 81).

The following are my observations about the descending ramus of the hypoglossal nerve and its connection with the cervical nerves [Figures 99-104].

After swabbing the point where it leaves the trunk with acetic acid or after having cautiously removed the neurilemma, it can always be seen that the ramus is connected through at least two roots with this trunk, one being thicker and leaving the trunk centrally and the other being much thinner and entering the trunk peripherally. Although it is rather easy to trace the course of the former for a certain distance up the trunk, its fibers then get so closely connected with those of the trunk that it is usually not possible to find out whether they belong to the roots of the hypoglossal itself or to the fibers of the cervical nerves which have merged further up with the trunk, or of the sympathetic or of the vagus nerve. Personally, I have seen only one case where that was possible. However, since it is well known that the relation of the trunk of the hypoglossal as well as that of the descending ramus

FIGURE 99

This figure shows a preparation—hard to define—of the connection between the hypoglossal (a) and the first cervical nerve (b). It deals mainly with the strand (f) which at first I thought represented the loop without end mentioned by Hyrtl, because in fact a distinct branch of the first cervical nerve (g) sometimes enters the trunk of the hypoglossal nerve. Finally, however, I arrived at the conclusion that (f) is a branch of a sympathetic plexus which spreads out between and together with the branches of the first cervical nerve; its one trunk is shown in (e). The strand (f) has already appeared in Figures 69 and 96 (k) and (g). It always exists and must not be confused with other fine fibers that ascend centrally along the hypoglossal nerve; in our case all of them seem to have merged in (g). Incidentally, it is also possible that this strand passes peripherally from the hypoglossal nerve into the first cervical nerve, and that it could spread out peripherally through one of the branches of the latter; but this could not be verified. This nerve is merely a portion of the main connecting branch (d) between the first cervical and the hypoglossal nerve which merges almost entirely with the hypoglossal nerve. (h) pictures a small strand of the first cervical nerve that merges with the hypoglossal nerve peripherally. (c) is the anastomosis between the first and the second cervical nerve.

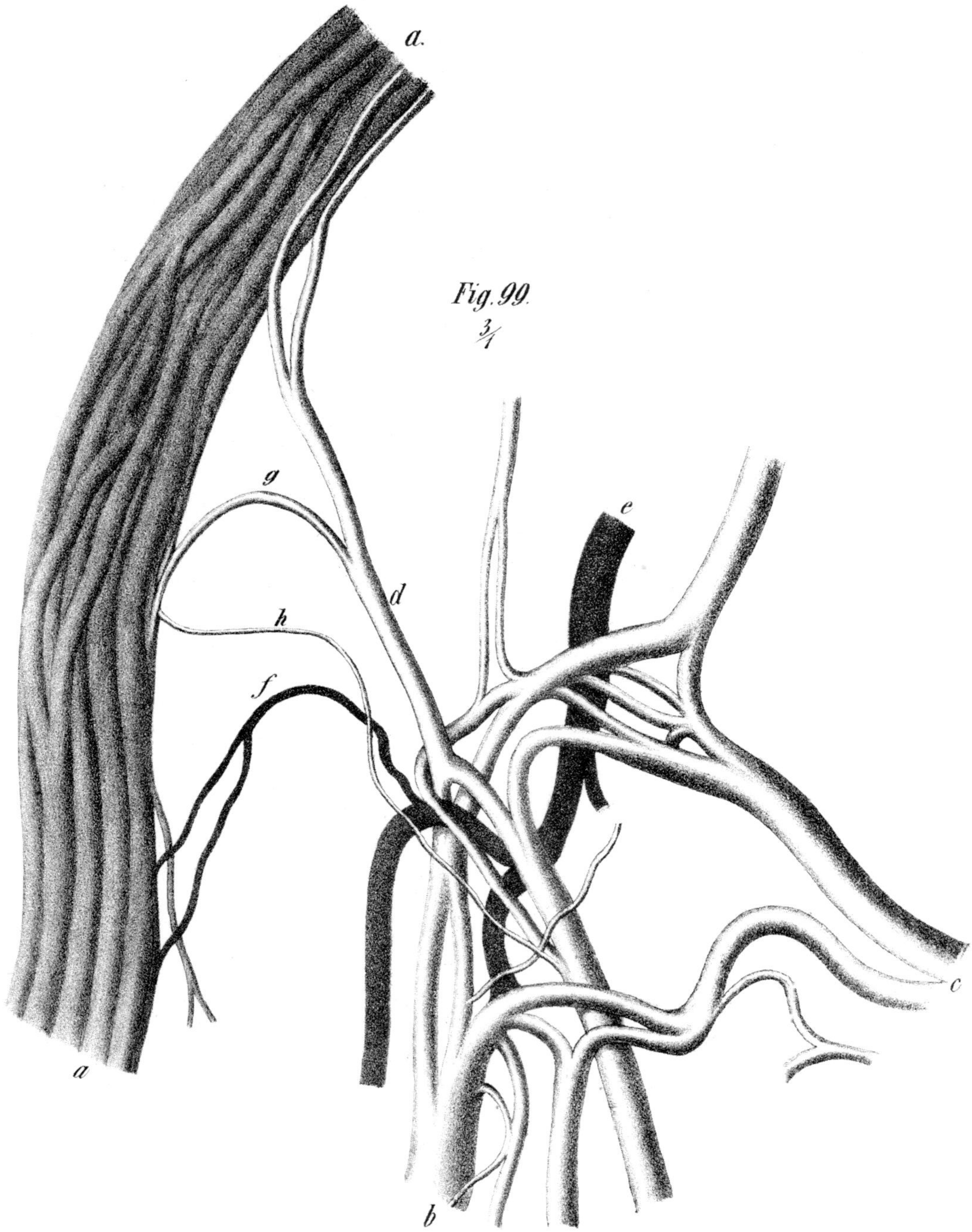

Fig. 99.
3/1

FIGURES 100 TO 104

These figures represent the well known ansa of the hypoglossal nerve between the latter and the second and third cervical nerves.

a hypoglossal nerve

b connecting branch of the first cervical nerve with the hypoglossal, which can sometimes be traced as far as the descending ramus of the hypoglossal nerve

dd second and third cervical nerves

cc a cut through the descending ramus of the hypoglossal nerve of which the central course has been omitted in order to save space

e portion of the descending ramus entering the hypoglossal nerve peripherally

f anastomosis between the descending ramus and the cervical nerve

Figure 101 shows just the trunk of the hypoglossal nerve (a) and the origin of its descending ramus from the cervical nerve (b).

Fig. 100.

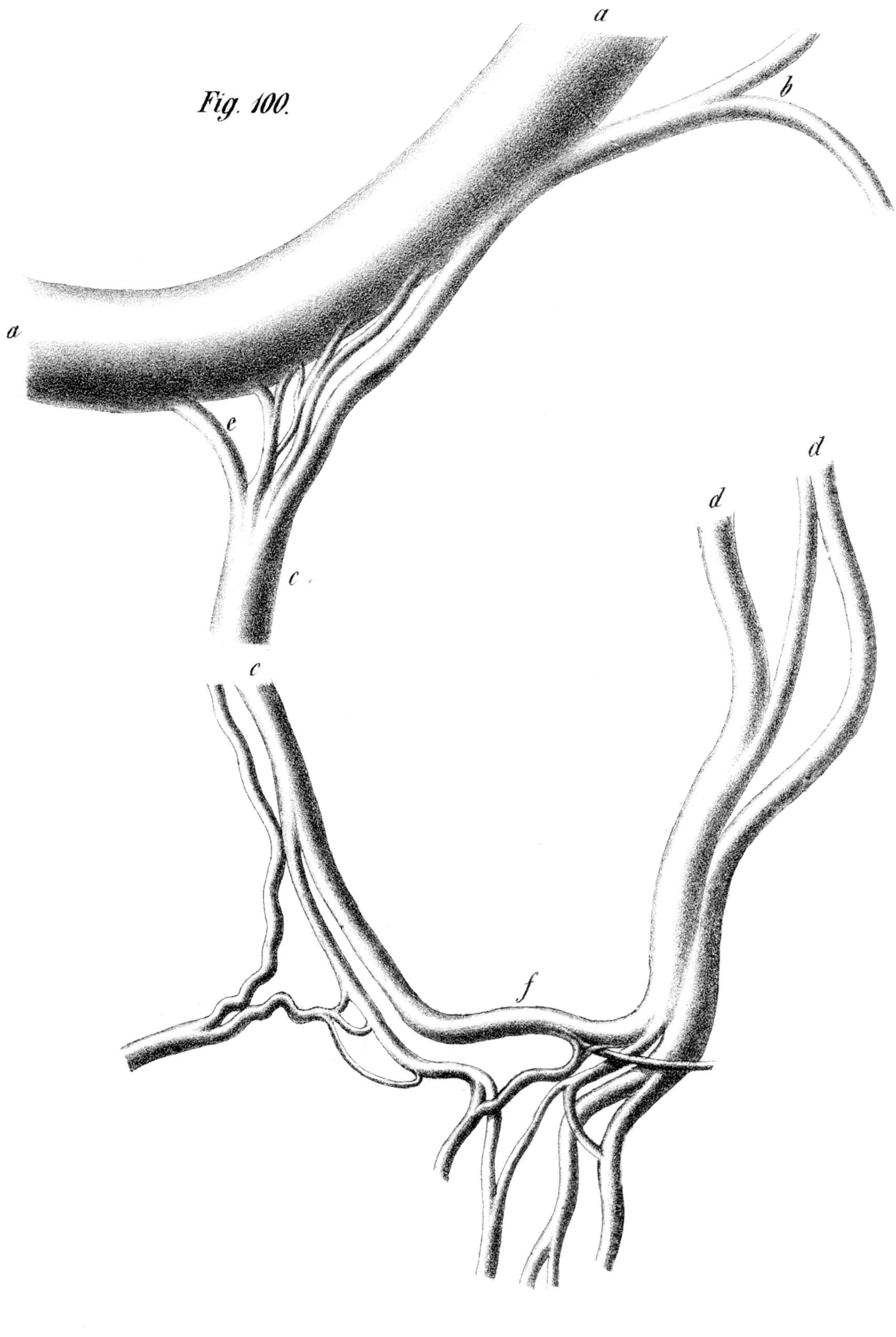

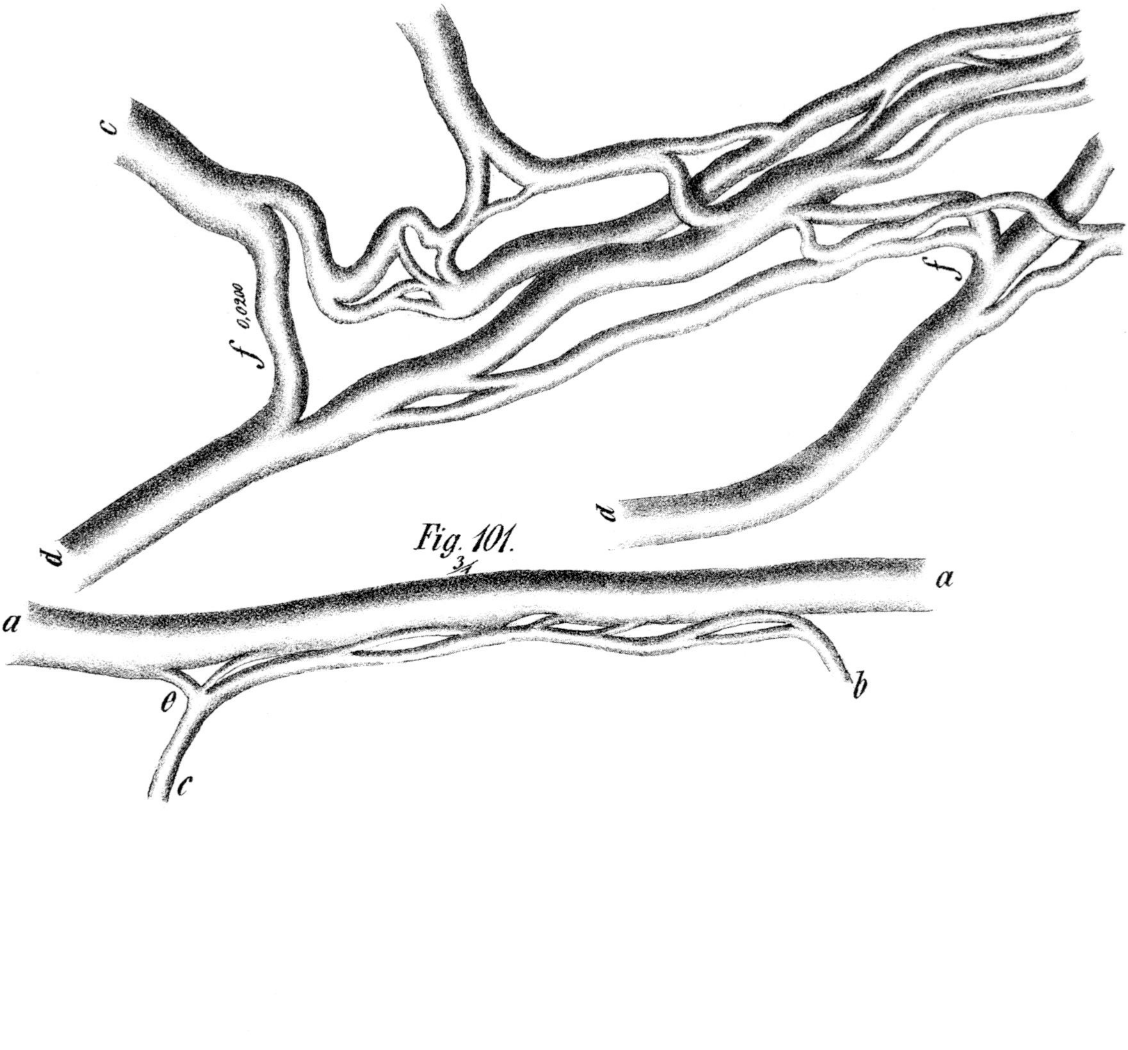

Fig. 101.
3/1

Fig. 102.

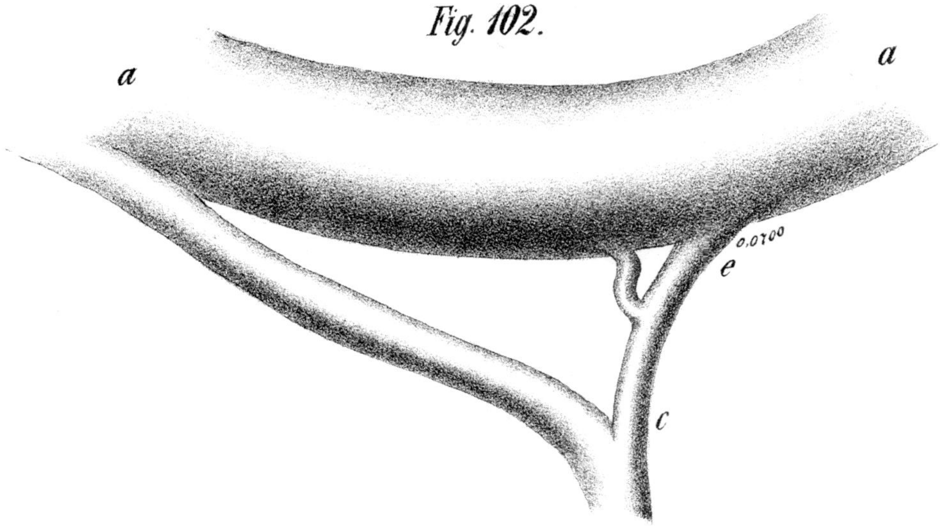

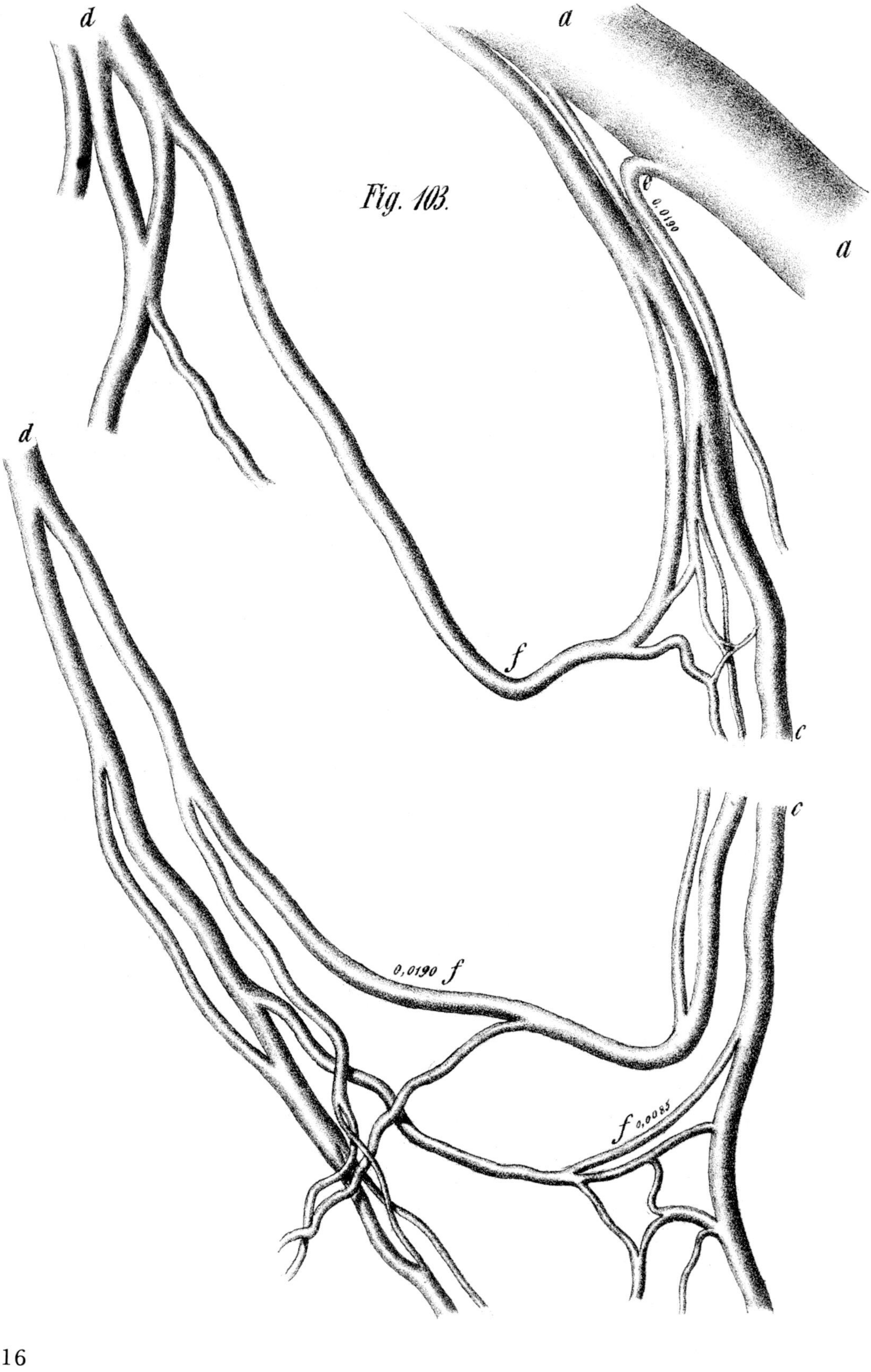

Fig. 103.

Fig. 104.

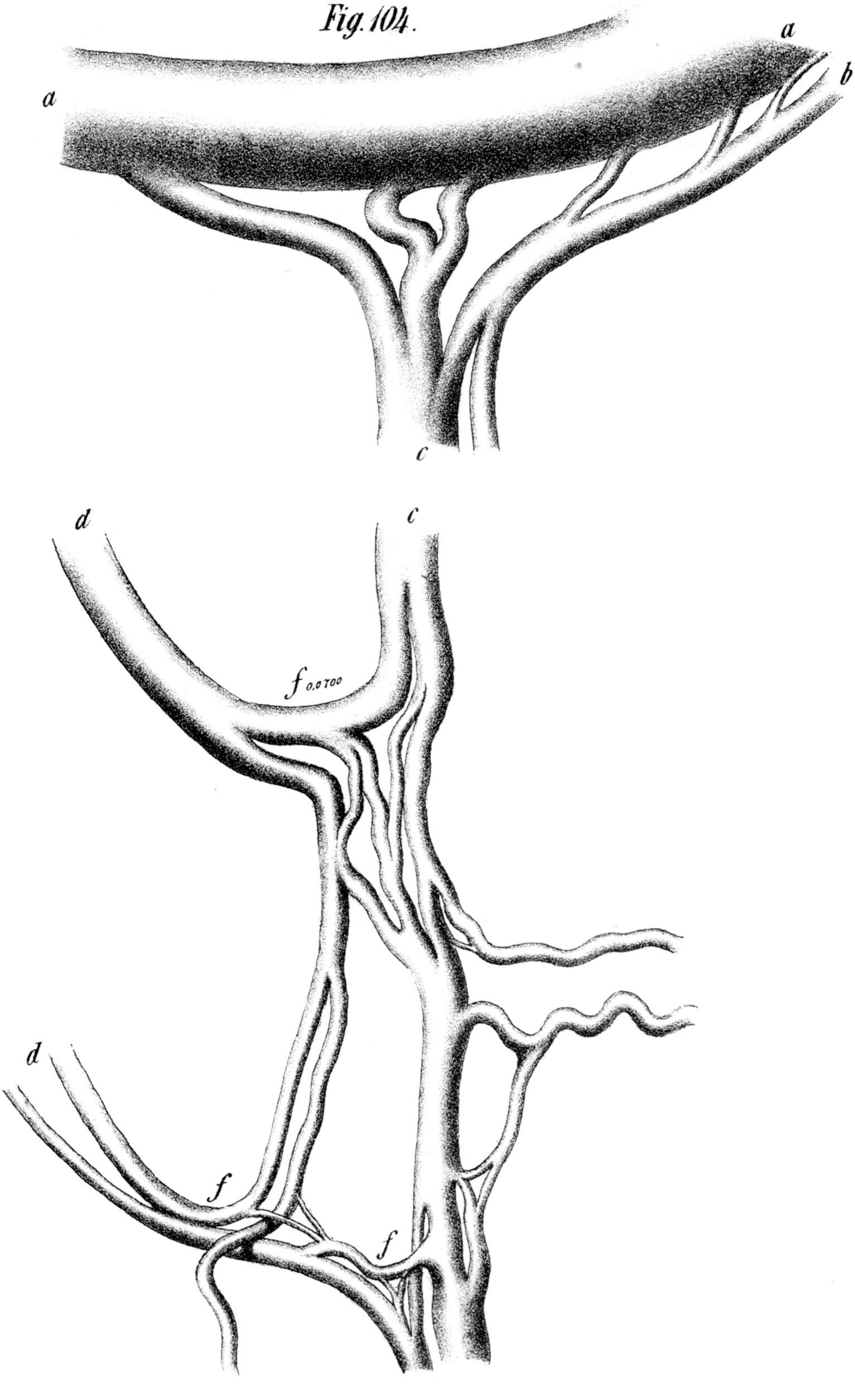

to the upper cervical nerves and the sympathetic nerve and particularly to the vagus varies greatly, I do not wish to deny that perhaps such isolated cases can shed some light on the origin of these stronger central roots of the descending ramus.

Although in such a case the descending ramus, if examined without special preparation and with the naked eye, seems to consist of just one nerve fascicle, if pressed between two slides or even better after treatment and clearing of the sheath with the help of acetic acid, it can be seen that it formed a plexus of long interchanging bundles, among which the small root running peripherally within the trunk can also be detected at its start though not for a very long stretch. Also, single nerves run into the surrounding area; but I cannot say exactly where they are going. However, finally when the descending ramus has for the most part descended to the intermediate tendon of the omohyoid muscle, it is divided into two parts which enter into the well known arc-shaped anastomosis with the ramus formed by the second and the third cervical nerve.

I said "by the second and the third cervical nerve" because never did I see, as Sappey claims to have seen, any nerve coming from the fourth cervical nerve participating in the formation of this anastomosis; on the other hand, I have sometimes seen three strands, one coming from the second, one from the third cervical nerve, and one from the branches of the respective nerves, and they form a small trunk which sometimes is divided on the way and also sends small fibers into the surrounding area. But in the end, when it approaches the anastomosis with the descending ramus, it always gets divided into two branches just like the latter. In this last respect Sappey's observation is right. The two upper or inner branches of those two nerves merge and form the anastomosis. The two lower or outer ones develop a small plexus, and from it those nerves originate that descend to the muscles.

I believe that I have given the important points of this anastomosis without going into complicated details that would apply to just one case at a time. The problem is not an easy one, neither with regard to the division of the descending ramus of the hypoglossal and the cervical nerve into an inner or outer ramus, nor in regard to the fact that the upper or inner branches not only merge, but also are involved in various ways in the small plexus. But they always form the anastomosis, and the question arises how to interpret this fact. As mentioned before, Volkmann offers a twofold explanation:

1. there are fibers inside the anastomosis which enter the trunk of the hypoglossal nerve peripherally

2. and fibers that run centrally within it and thus form the end-loop.

Arnold is undecided, while Sappey accepts only the first explanation. It seems clear that in order to come to a decision one should be able to say that the fibers that form the anastomosis are more numerous than those which come from the trunk and enter the hypoglossal nerve peripherally. If this is the case, the remaining portion must run inside the central root, and that means indeed that it forms a central loop between cervical and hypoglossal nerve, or between the cervical cord and the medulla oblongata.

Unfortunately, my measurements with Schick's micrometric screw did not produce a decisive result because it was not possible to use the screw without applying pressure, and this treatment may have caused discrepancies that in reality did not exist. This seems to me all the more probable since the peripheral root at the hypoglossal nerve almost always measured 0.0130 mm:* because of the thickness of the hypoglossal nerve the pressure caused less change here than in the anastomosis where the results of the measurements varied to a greater extent.

Incidentally, I do not believe that what we see here is such an anastomosis without end, but simply a very strange course of fibers of the cervical nerves heading upward in the descending ramus and then peripherally in the hypoglossal nerve. If, however, more fascicles should really be contained in the anastomosis than in the root of the descending ramus running peripherally, it is quite possible that this greater number runs peripherally somewhere higher in the trunk of the hypoglossal nerve or of the cranial nerves, and therefore does not represent a loop between two central points.

I did not study the course of those nerves which come from the anastomotic plexus at the omohyoid muscle and therefore cannot state whether they go to the cervical nerves and if they do go there (which they doubtlessly do) whether they originate from the cervical nerves or from the descending ramus of the hypoglossal nerve; nor can I say where the fibers of the latter go if they do not run into the muscles. This can only be determined by an experiment like that of Volkmann, since the two nerves undergo an exchange in the manner of a plexus. I would like to add the fact that I seemed to detect at the small plexus mentioned above some sympathetic nerves that came from the adjacent area and appeared to be involved in the process.

*[Bischoff uses the abbreviation "mass." here, which we cannot translate except as "millimeters." *Ed.*]

Finally, the hypoglossal nerve forms the well known anastomosis with the lingual nerve at the point where both nerves reach the margin of the tongue [Figures 105-109]. No one as yet has made a detailed description of the kind of connection between those two nerves with the exception of Arnold, who claims that the connecting branches originating from the lingual nerve seem to come from the maxillary ganglion or to go in the sheath of the lingual nerve from the hypoglossal nerve to the maxillary ganglion. The anastomosis on the other hand is quite simple. Although it looks like an arc-shaped transition of fibers of the two nerves into each other, it consists merely of a plexus-like connection of both nerves, all fibers of which leave again peripherally. Only once did I examine a preparation that seemed to contain an anastomosis without end; but here, too, it cannot be determined whether the fibers of this anastomosis leave either the lingual nerve or the hypoglossal peripherally at a higher point.

Professor Luschka has furnished a special description of the hypoglossal nerve (*Müller's Archiv,* 1856, p. 62) which also includes the examination of its anastomoses with other nerves. Luschka mentions first a connection between the superior cervical ganglion of the sympathetic and the trunk of the hypoglossal nerve 6 mm. below the hypoglossal canal, and he states that it is anatomically impossible to decide whether it goes from the sympathetic to the hypoglossal nerve or vice versa. As far as the descending ramus is concerned, he claims that it always originates from the first or from the first and second cervical nerve and has nothing to do with the hypoglossal itself. In addition he confirms the existence of a few small strands running from one of the three cervical nerves toward the central end of the hypoglossal nerve; those, however, leave the latter for a spreading out peripherally. Luschka does not mention at all the connection of the descending hypoglossal ramus with the anterior ramus of the second and third cervical nerve in the so-called ansa hypoglossal, nor the peripheral course of some fibers at the origin of the descending ramus in the trunk of the hypoglossal nerve; consequently he does not mention Volkmann's work, since as we said earlier, he concludes that the descending ramus comes entirely from the cervical nerves. According to Luschka there is not even a trace of a connection between the vagus and hypoglossal nerve, for the connection of the small strands that go from the vagus to the hypoglossal nerve, then immediately leave the latter again and return into the vagus, only appear to be one. However, Luschka emphasizes the connection of the hypoglossal nerve with strands coming from the lingual nerve of the trigeminal and from the submaxillary ganglion close to the tongue. He says that a portion of those strands makes that connection and always runs cen-

FIGURES 105 TO 107

Figures 105 to 107 picture the equally well known anastomosis between the hypoglossal and lingual nerves. After joining, the branches spread out further peripherally in a different sequence.

Fig. 105.

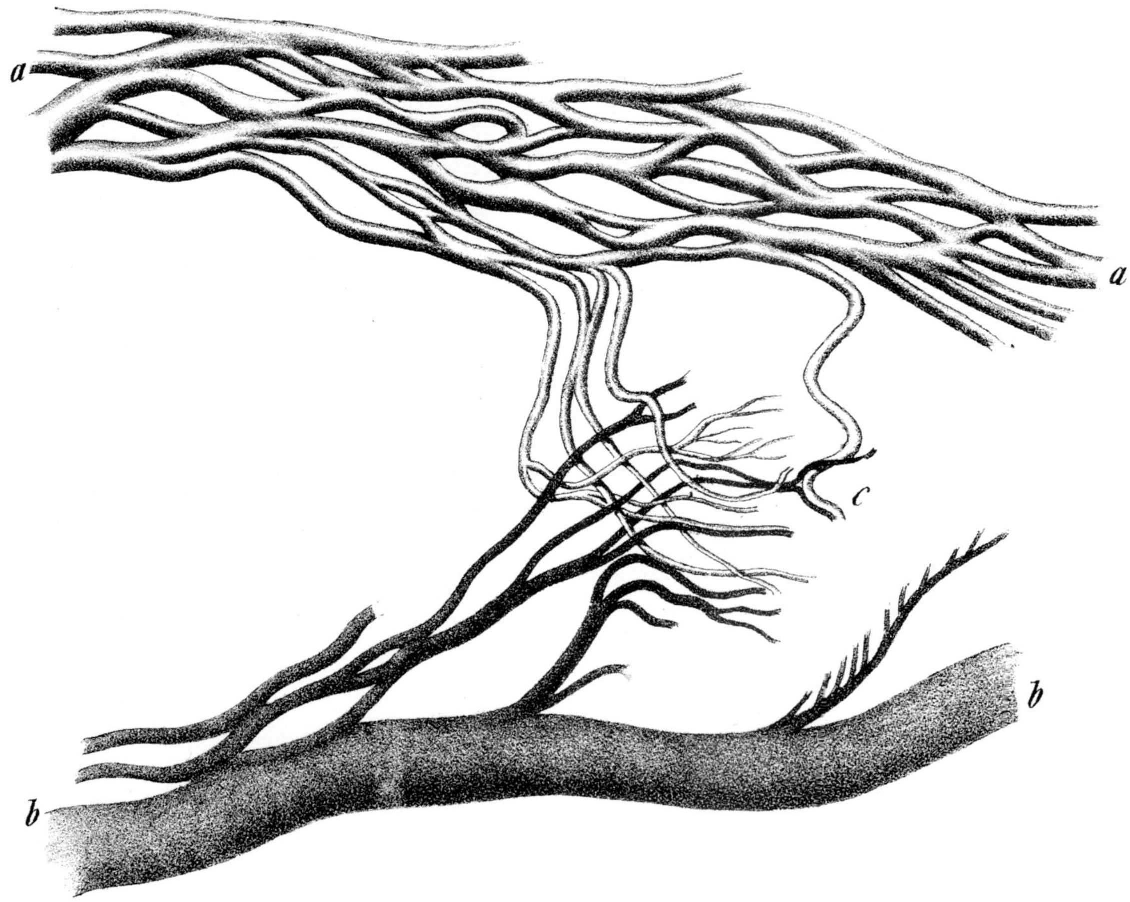

Fig. 106.

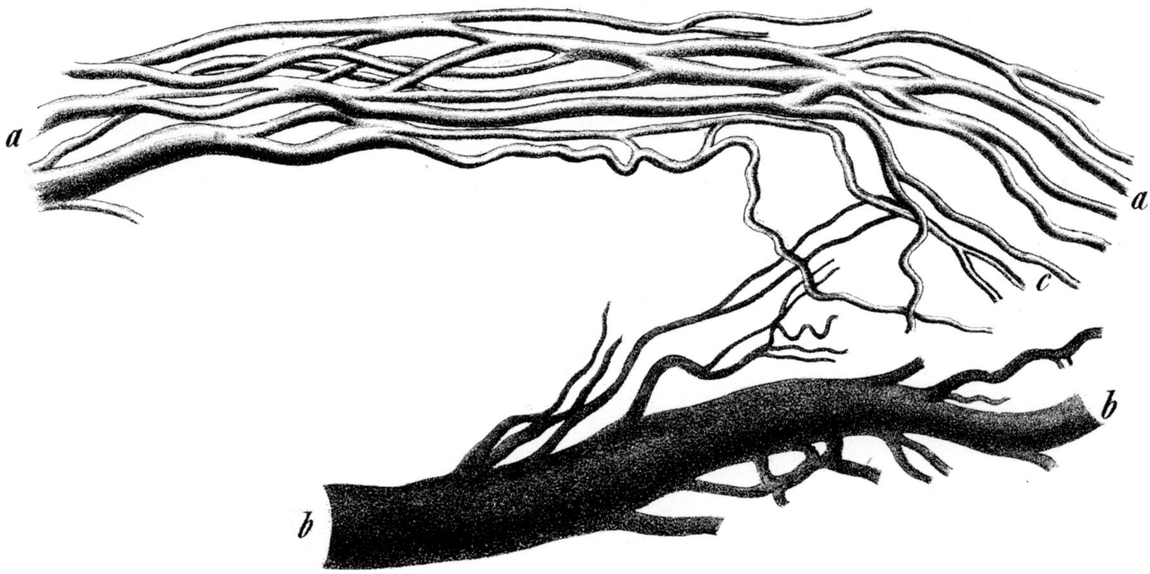

Fig. 107.

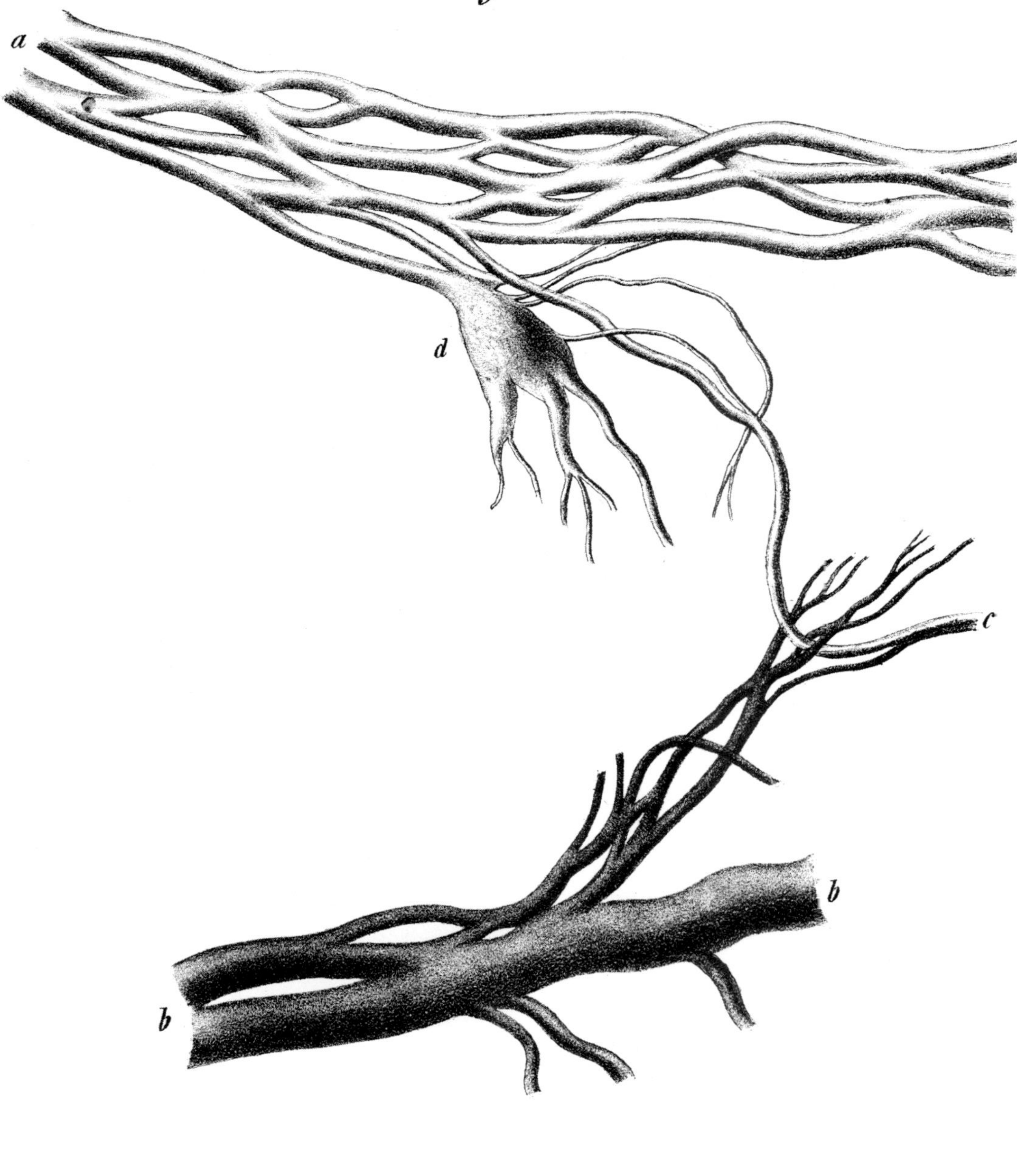

FIGURE 108-109

This seems to be the only figure that shows a so-called loop without end. But it may have found its peripheral end at some other spot. In spite of frequent experiments I never found it again at this particular spot.

a lingual nerve

b hypoglossal nerve

c anastomosis between (a) and (b)

d lingual ganglion

Fig. 108.

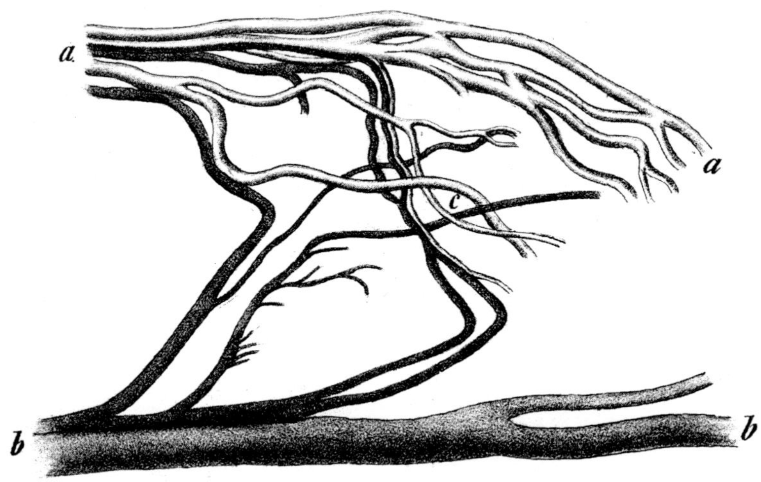

Fig. 109.

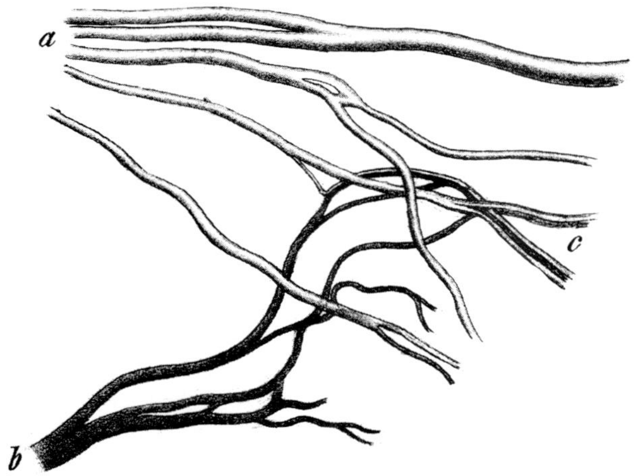

trally toward the root of the hypoglossal nerve. Supposedly their importance lies in their sensory function, and they leave the trunk of the hypoglossal nerve again to cause spreading out at the periphery mainly as nerves of the occipital bone and as nerves to the circular sinus of the foramen magnum.

Results

1. No anastomoses exist between the upper three [I, II, and VIII—*ed.*] sensory nerves and any other nerve. Even the one between the acoustic and the facial nerve is only an apparent one brought about by the so-called nervus intermedius which, although it belongs for the most part to the facial nerve, partially belongs to the acoustic nerve. [Very confusing, but this is an important connection. *Ed.*]

2. The three oculomotor nerves do not enter into an anastomosis with any cranial nerve except the trochlear nerve, which often takes in a small strand of the ophthalmic branch of the trigeminal nerve.

3. The tentorial nerve of the cerebellum is a branch not of the trochlear nerve but of the ophthalmic ramus of the trigeminal nerve.

4. The anastomosis between the lacrimal (V^1) and the zygmatico-temporal branch of (V^2) is nothing but a passage of fibers of the latter to those of the former peripherally mainly into the lacrimal gland.

5. The same is true of the superior and the inferior trochlear nerve branches of the fifth. They merely lie alongside each other and have a common peripheral course.

6. The so-called vidian nerve contains a thread of the internal carotid nerve going to the sphenopalatine nerve (the greater deep petrosal nerve) and a connection between the ganglion just mentioned and the geniculate ganglion of the facial nerve (the greater superficial petrosal nerve), the fibers of which cannot be traced beyond those ganglia. In its entire course the vidian is more a plexus of nerves than a single or double nerve.

7. The chorda tympani is in its strongest part a branch of the seventh nerve, and most of its fibers come from the central part of this nerve; but it cannot be traced to another origin. However, usually

the tympanic nerve gives off at its point of origin a strand that runs peripherally into the facial nerve; the origin of this nerve most probably lies in the otic ganglion. Fibers run peripherally as well as centrally from this ganglion into the chorda. Furthermore, during its course alongside the lingual nerve the latter merges so often with the fibers of this nerve that one can by no means be sure, but only assume, that roots pass from it into the submaxillary ganglion.

8. The auricular branch of the vagus nerve [Arnold's] varies greatly in its course. In the first place it may not exist at all. Usually it originates from the vagus and the glossopharyngeal nerve, but at this point of origin it also has fibers that enter those nerves peripherally. Frequently it consists of two fascicles, of which one probably originates from the small thread that passes from the trunk of the facial into the auricular nerve. Often it sends a small twig peripherally into the facial nerve, and sometimes it merges peripherally with the facial nerve. Finally it also happens occasionally that there is no connection whatsoever with the facial nerve.

9. The anastomosis between the facial and the superficial temporal branch of the third branch of the trigeminal nerve contains only fibers that run from the latter peripherally alongside the branches of the facial nerve. The same is true of the anastomoses between the infraorbital and the mental nerve and the branches of the trigeminal nerve.

10. The tympanic plexus, or Jacobson's anastomosis, is not only a broadening of the tympanic nerve from the glossopharyngeal, but it is a genuine anastomosis, a plexus between the otic ganglion, the petrosal ganglion and the internal carotid plexus, from which fibers also pass peripherally into the glossopharyngeal. Those nerves that run from the plexus to the Eustachian tube are derived from the tympanic nerve as well as from the lesser superficial petrosal and also the sympathetic nerve. A small microscopic ganglion almost always appears at the small strand going toward the oval window.

11. All authors with the exception of Beck speak of an anastomosis between the lesser superficial petrosal and the geniculate ganglion formed by a small artery, as Beck rightly states. [Wrong, according to Gray's. *Ed.*]

12. The posterior roots of the first cervical nerve are not strictly separated from the roots and the trunk of the accessory nerve, but in reality they are derived from the former and also merge with the trunk of the accessory—from which, however, they probably separate again at the end.

13. It cannot justly be said that the accessory nerve in the jugular foramen is strictly separated from the vagus nerve and its jugular ganglion. There are two possibilities; either some of its roots are involved in the formation of this ganglion or, what is more likely, some small strands of the vagus coming from this ganglion join the accessory before the latter is divided into an inner and an outer branch.

14. The anastomosis between the accessory and the third cervical nerve possibly contains an anastomosis without end.

15. The anastomosis between the hypoglossal and the first cervical nerve has various aspects. In the first place it is only an apparent one, which is formed by a sympathetic nerve. It seems that a central anastomosis without end exists sometimes. A constant peripheral anastomosis cannot always be traced to the descending ramus.

*
16. The anastomosis from the hypoglossal to the vagus, which is usually mentioned, is merely an apparent one. But there are several fine connections between those two nerves which mostly run from the vagus to the hypoglossal.

* 17. Fibers are found in the ansa hypoglassi between the descending ramus of the hypoglossal and the second and third cervical nerve which continue their course peripherally from the point of origin of the descending ramus in the hypoglossal nerve. This fact indicated that they are derived from the cervical nerves. I continue to be doubtful with regard to the question whether this ansa contains fibers that run centrally from the above-mentioned point of origin of the descending ramus within the hypoglossal nerve and therefore represent a loop without end.

18. The well known connection between a branch of the hypoglossal and a branch of the lingual nerve close to the tongue usually is nothing but a close peripheral course of the fibers of both branches. Occasionally, an apparent loop without end can be detected.

* [Bischoff completely contradicts himself here. Having demonstrate the anatomical connections by dissection, he seems to forget he did it! *Ed.*]

Summary of Findings and Their Clinical Importance

BY ERNEST SACHS, JR., M.D.

The anatomists in France, England, America, and particularly in Germany in the eighteenth and nineteenth centuries speculated from their dissections that there were connections between various cranial nerves. Bischoff brought together in his monograph the conflicting theories, arguments, and findings of the most prominent workers in his field. He settled many of the arguments by his meticulous dissections, and was painstakingly thorough, self-critical, and honest in his conclusions. He showed beyond any reasonable doubt that there are innumerable connections and pathways between the trigeminal, facial, nervus intermedius, vestibular, glossopharyngeal, vagus, spinal accessory, hypoglossal, and upper cervical nerves, as well as the sympathetic and parasympathetic nerves.

The importance of this from the clinical standpoint is of great significance in undertaking analysis and explanation of many of the "atypical" pain syndromes about the face, head, and neck. Neurologists, neurosurgeons, and otolaryngologists in particular are frequently confronted with syndromes difficult to diagnose and treat about the face, head, ears, pharynx, and sinuses. Ramsay Hunt, J. G. Sluder, Wilfred Harris, F. W. L. Kerr, B. T. Horton, and many others have postulated all sorts of mechanisms for these syndromes of facial pain. Some of the anatomical substrate seems to have been lost in the last hundred years, so that gross anatomy books and neuroanatomy texts have not addressed themselves to these little connecting "threads and strands" to which Bischoff paid so much attention.

At times, if one reads the texts carefully—a laborious task even when translated into as fluent English as possible—Bischoff seems to be ambivalent about his findings. Whereas his text and dissections clearly convinced him of anastomosis in certain places, he seems to back off from what appeared to him a too radical assumption in his "Results"—which was written after the original paper won the prize.

Bischoff realized and clearly stated (pages 10 and 80) that the axones of one nerve did not actually enter into those of another, but just as no one will doubt the connection of the lingual nerve to the seventh via the chorda tympani, so also, many of the connections he showed were matters of the fibers of one nerve leaving it and traveling along with another one. This of course leads to the important possibility that a lesion affecting one nerve at a given spot will also affect another at that spot also. Many of the connections shown by Bischoff help explain the perseveration or loss of sensation in the face, tongue, eyes, and ears when the lesions observed would lead one to think such a function would or would not be affected.

The myriads of interconnecting strands between the fifth, seventh, eight, ninth, tenth, eleventh, twelfth, and C1, 2, and 3 nerves may help explain many syndromes of head and face pain and ear, throat, Eustachian tube, and neck pain, which are so hard to treat when involved by malignant disease or functional imbalance such as cluster headache and atypical facial neuralgia. The latter term, coined by Glaser in 1928, is an unfortunately negative "nondiagnosis." It merely means a syndrome not typical of tic douloureux. It may be entirely typical of some other disorder or disorders, the etiology of which we do not yet understand.

Pain during Bell's palsy, residual facial sensation after the trigeminal nerve has been cut, taste and tear preservation (Schwartz and Weddell, and Sachs) after the facial nerve has been severed, and pain in the ear from cancer after the fifth, seventh, nervus intermedius, ninth, tenth, C1 and 2 have been severed, may be explained by these connections between the cranial nerves.

Conclusion

Bischoff's work has been lost sight of, and its rediscovery deserves examination and consideration in the diagnosis and treatment of syndromes of the head, face, and neck.

Notes about Bischoff's References

Arnold, Friederick, 1803–1867. *Handbuch der Anatomie,* 1851.

Beck, Thomas Snow, 1814–1867. *Über die Verbindung des Sehn-nerven mit dem Augen- und Nasen-Knoten,* Heidelberg, 1847.

———*Anat. Unter. über das VII und IX Hirnnerven paar.*

Bidder, Heinrich Friederick, 1810, 1894. Described the lesser superficial petrosal nerve with Volkmann.

Bischoff, Theodore Ludwig Wilhelm, 1806–1882. Professor and Head of the Anatomical Institute in Munich. Father of Ernst Philip Eduard Bischoff. *Commentatio de Nervi accessori. Anat. et Phys.,* 1832.

Bock, August Carl, 1782-1833. German anatomist.

Boehmer. De Nona pari nervi cerebri. In *Ludwig's Script. Neurol.,* I, p. 294.

Boyer, Alexis, Baron de, 1757–1833. French surgeon.

Breschet, Gilbert, 1784–1845. *Recherches anatomique et physiologique sur l'organe de l'ouie et sur l'audition dans l'homme et les animaux Vertèbres,* Paris, 1836.

Caldani, Leopoldo Mario Antonio, 1725–1813. Professor of Anatomy in Bologna. A teacher of Galvani.

Chaussier, François, 1746–1828. Parisian surgeon and anatomist.

Cloquet, Jules Hippolyte, 1787–1840. Described the nasopalatine ganglion in 1820.

Cruveillhier, Jean, 1791-1874. French pathologist.

Cusco, G., *Anatomie,* II, Paris, 1853.

Guidi, Guido (Vidius), 1508-1569. Described the Vidian nerve.

Haller, Albrecht Von. *Elementa physiologicae carporis humani. Tomus quartus cerebrum Nervi. musculi.* Lausanne, Francisci Grasset, 1762.

Hirschfeld, Ludwig. *Neurologie et Iconographie du Systeme Nerveux et des organes des Sens de l'homme,* Paris, 1853. 92 plates in color.

Hirzel, *Zeitschrift für Physiologie,* I, p. 228.

Hyrtl, Josef, 1810–1894. Eminent anatomist. A Hungarian, Professor of Anatomy at Prague at age 26. Eight years later returned to Vienna as Professor of Anatomy. *Lehrbuch der Anatomie des Menschen,* Vienna, 1862, and *Nat. Hist. Review,* January 1862.

Jacobsen, Ludwig Levin, 1783–1843. Worked out the origin and course of the tympanic nerve and plexus, and the connection with the carotid plexus which bears his name.

Kölliker, Rudolph Albert von, 1817–1905. Born in Zurich. Professor at Wurzburg, 1847. *Gewebelehre,* 4th ed.

Krause, Karl Friederick Theodore, 1797–1868.

Kronenberg, Henricus, 1813. *Plexum nervorum structura et Virtutes,* Berlin, 1836.

Langenbeck, Conrad Johann, 1776–1851.

Lauth, Thomas, 1758–1826. Strasbourg anatomist and surgeon.

Lobstein, Johann Georg Christian Friedrick Martin, 1777–1835. First Professor of Pathology at Strasbourg. Wrote a 2-volume *Treatise on Pathological Anatomy,* Paris, 1829–33.

Longet, François-Achille, 1811–1871. Wrote a beautiful anatomy and physiology of the nervous system of man and animals, *Anatomie und Physiologie des Nervensystems,* 2 vols., Paris, 1842.

Luschka, Hubert von, 1820–1875. Celebrated German anatomist. Described the foramina with his name, in *Müller's Archiv,* 1856.

Martin, Henry Austin, 1824–1884. American surgeon.

Mayer, August Franz Joseph Carl, 1787–1865. Studied trophic disturbances of the eye after trigeminal section, *Acta nat. Curios.* XVI, 1833.

Meckel, Johann Friedrick, the Elder, 1724–1774. *Tractus Anatomico-physiologicus de quinto pare nervorum cerebri,* Göttingen, A. Vandenhoeck, 1748. This was Meckel's graduation thesis, a classical description of the sphenopalatine ganglion that bears his name, and the dural space lodging the Gasserian ganglion and the motor roots. See Saunders and Sachs, below.

Müller, Johannes, 1801–1858. One of the greatest German anatomists. Founder and editor of *Müller's Archiv.*

Murray, Johannes Andreas, 1740–1797.

Pappenheim, Samuel Moritz, 1811–1882. Of Breslau. Studied the nerves to the cornea. *Gewebelehre des Gehorgans.*

Ribes, François J., 1800–1867. Memoire sur quelques parties d'oreille interne, *Rev. Med. franc. et etrang.,* 12:260, 801–23.

Rudiger. Associate of Professor Dr. T. L. W. Bischoff.

Sappey, Marie Philbert Constant, 1810–1896. *Anatomie Descriptive,* 1852.

Scarpa, Antonio, 1747–1832. *Tabulae neurologicae, ad illustrandum historiam anatomicam, cardiacorum nervorum. Noni nervorum cerebri, glossopharyngaei, et pharyngaei ex octavo cerebri.* A skillful artist and one of the best of the medical men who illustrated their own books.

Sommering, Samuel Thomas, 1755–1830. *Das Sehorgan.*

Spencer, Oliver. *Edin. Med. and Surg. Journal,* 1842, p. 397.

Swan, Joseph, 1791–1874. Wrote a treatise on disease and injuries of the nerves and studied nerve regeneration, London, 1824.

Tiedmann, Friedrick, 1781–1861. Zeitschrift V. p. 177.

Valentin, Gabriel Gustav. 1810–1883. *Hirn und Nervenlehre,* 1841.

Varrentrapp, Johann Georgius, 1809–1886. *Observationes Anatomiae, Nerve Sympathia,* Frankfurtia, Parte Cephalica, No. 183, 38 pp., with 4 tables.

Volkmann, Alfred Wilhelm, 1800–1887. *Müller's Archiv,* 1840, p. 520.

Willis, Sir Thomas, 1621–1675. Great British anatomist who described the arterial anastomotic circle that bears his name.

Wrisberg, Heinrich August, 1739-1808. *Observatione anatomicae de quinto pare nervorum, encephali.* Göttingen, J. C. Dietrich, 1777. Wrisberg, Professor of Anatomy at Göttingen, is remembered for his discovery of the nervus intermedius between the seventh and eighth cranial nerves.

Modern Works Cited

Cooper, D. W., and Cavicke, D. C., Primary juvenile otalgia. Report of a case with surgical cure, *J. Neurosurg.*, 1963, 20:895–98.

Furlow, L. T., Tic douloureux of the nervus intermedius (so-called idiopathic geniculate neuralgia), *JAMA*, 1942, 199:255–59.

Glaser, M. A., Atypical neuralgia, so-called. A critical analysis of 143 cases. *Arch. Neurol. Psychiat.*, Chicago, 1928, 20:537-58.

Harris, W., *Neuritis and Neuralgia*, New York, Oxford University Press, 1926, p. 432.

Horton, B. T., MacLean, A. R., and Craig, W. M., A new syndrome of vascular headache. Results of treatment with histamine; preliminary report, *Proc. Mayo Clinic*, 1939, 14:257–60.

Hunt, J. R., Geniculate Neuralgia (Neuralgia of the nervus facialis). A further contribution to the sensory system of the facial nerve and its neuralgic conditions, *Arch. Neurol. Psychiat.*, Chicago, 1937, 37:253–85.

Kerr, F. W. L., Facial, vagal and glossopharyngeal nerves in the cat, *Arch. Neurol. Psychiat.*, Chicago, 1962, 6:264–81.

Penfield, W., and McNaughton, F., Dural headache and innervation of the dura mater, *Arch. Neurol. Psychiat.*, Chicago, 1940, 44:43–75.

Rhoton, A. L., Kobayashi, S., and Hollinshead, W. H., Nervus intermedius, *J. Neurosurg.*, 1968, 29:609–18.

Sachs, E., Jr., The role of the nervus intermedius in facial neuralgia. Report of four cases with observations on the pathways for taste, lacrimation, and pain in the face, *J. Neurosurg.*, 1968, 28:54–60.

Saunders, R. L., and Sachs, E., Jr., Relation of the accessory rootlets of the trigeminal nerve to its motor root. *J. Neurosurg.*, 1970, 33:317-24.

Schwartz, H. G., and Weddell, G., Observations on the pathways transmitting the sensation of taste, *Brain*, 1938, 61:99–115.

Sluder, J. G., Headaches and eye disorders of nasal origin, St. Louis, C. V. Mosby, 1918, 272 pp.

White, J. C., and Sweet, W., *Pain. Its Mechanisms and Neurosurgical Control*, Springfield, Illinois, C. C. Thomas, 1955, 736 pp.

Wilson, A. A., Geniculate neuralgia. Report of a case relieved by intracranial section of the nerve of Wrisberg, *J. Neurosurg.*, 1950, 7:473–81.

Reference Books

Garrison's History of Neurology. Revised and enlarged with a bibliography of classical, original, and standard works in "Neurology," ed. McHenry, Lawrence C., Jr., Springfield, Illinois, C. C. Thomas, 1969, 552 pp.

Gray's Anatomy, 35th British edition, ed. Warwick, Roger, and Williams, Peter L., Philadelphia, W. B. Saunders, 1973, 1471 pp.

History of Medicine, Mettler, C. C., and Mettler, Fred A., Jr., Philadelphia, Blakiston, 1947, 1215 pp.

Anatomy of the Human Body, Lockhard, R. D., Hamilton, G. F., and Fyfe, F. W., Philadelphia, J. B. Lippincott, 1965, 3rd printing, 705 pp.

A Medical Bibliography (Garrison and Morton). Annotated checklist of texts illustrating the history of medicine, Morton, Leslie, T., Philadelphia, J. B. Lippincott, 1970, 3rd edition, 552 pp.